Penile, Urethral, and Scrotal Cancer

Editor

PHILIPPE E. SPIESS

UROLOGIC CLINICS
OF NORTH AMERICA

www.urologic.theclinics.com

Consulting Editor
SAMIR S. TANEJA

November 2016 • Volume 43 • Number 4

ELSEVIER

1600 John F. Kennedy Boulevard • Suite 1800 • Philadelphia, Pennsylvania, 19103-2899

http://www.theclinics.com

UROLOGIC CLINICS OF NORTH AMERICA Volume 43, Number 4
November 2016 ISSN 0094-0143, ISBN-13: 978-0-323-47696-6

Editor: Kerry Holland
Developmental Editor: Alison Swety

Urologic Clinics of North America (ISSN 0094-0143) is published quarterly by Elsevier Inc., 360 Park Avenue South, New York, NY 10010-1710. Months of issue are February, May, August, and November. Business and Editorial Offices: 1600 John F. Kennedy Blvd., Suite 1800, Philadelphia, PA 19103-2899. Periodicals postage paid at New York, NY and additional mailing offices. Subscription prices are $360.00 per year (US individuals), $660.00 per year (US institutions), $415.00 per year (Canadian individuals), $825.00 per year (Canadian institutions), $515.00 per year (foreign individuals), and $825.00 per year (foreign institutions). Foreign air speed delivery is included in all *Clinics* subscription prices. All prices are subject to change without notice. **POSTMASTER:** Send address changes to *Urologic Clinics of North America*, Elsevier Health Sciences Division, Subscription Customer Service, 3251 Riverport Lane, Maryland Heights, MO 63043. **Customer Service: 1-800-654-2452 (US). From outside the United States, call 1-314-447-8871. Fax: 1-314-447-8029. E-mail: JournalsCustomerServiceusa@elsevier.com (for print support)** and **JournalsOnlineSupport-usa@elsevier.com (for online support)**.

Reprints. For copies of 100 or more, of articles in this publication, please contact the Commercial Reprints Department, Elsevier Inc., 360 Park Avenue South, New York, New York 10010-1710. Tel.: 212-633-3874; Fax: 212-633-3820; E-mail: reprints@elsevier.com.

Urologic Clinics of North America is covered in MEDLINE/PubMed (*Index Medicus*), *Excerpta Medica, Current Contents/Clinical Medicine, Science Citation Index,* and *ISI/BIOMED.*

PROGRAM OBJECTIVE

The goal of *Urologic Clinics of North America* is to keep practicing urologists and urology residents up to date with current clinical practice in urology by providing timely articles reviewing the state of the art in patient care.

TARGET AUDIENCE

Practicing urologists, urology residents and other health care professionals practicing in the discipline of urology.

LEARNING OBJECTIVES

Upon completion of this activity, participants will be able to:

1. Review potential vaccinations for and management approaches to penile cancer.
2. Discuss management strategies for urethral cancers.
3. Recognize updates in the pathogenesis and evaluation of primary scrotal cancer.

ACCREDITATION

The Elsevier Office of Continuing Medical Education (EOCME) is accredited by the Accreditation Council for Continuing Medical Education (ACCME) to provide continuing medical education for physicians.

The EOCME designates this enduring material for a maximum of 15 *AMA PRA Category 1 Credit*(s)™. Physicians should claim only the credit commensurate with the extent of their participation in the activity.

All other health care professionals requesting continuing education credit for this enduring material will be issued a certificate of participation.

DISCLOSURE OF CONFLICTS OF INTEREST

The EOCME assesses conflict of interest with its instructors, faculty, planners, and other individuals who are in a position to control the content of CME activities. All relevant conflicts of interest that are identified are thoroughly vetted by EOCME for fair balance, scientific objectivity, and patient care recommendations. EOCME is committed to providing its learners with CME activities that promote improvements or quality in healthcare and not a specific proprietary business or a commercial interest.

The planning committee, staff, authors and editors listed below have identified no financial relationships or relationships to products or devices they or their spouse/life partner have with commercial interest related to the content of this CME activity:

Johnathan Beilan, MD; Michael Bickell, DO; Matt Broggi, MSc; Rafael Carrion, MD; Juanita Crook, MD, FRCPC; Gregory J. Diorio, DO; Anjali Fortna; Paul K. Hegarty, MB BCh BAO, Mch, FRCSI, FRCS (Urol); Kerry Holland; S. Horenblas, MD, PhD, FEBU; Jonathan H. Huang, MD; Wassim Kassouf, MD, CM, FRCS(C); Indu Kumari; Tharani Mahesan, MBBS, BSc, MRCS; Viraj A. Master, MD, PhD; S. Minhas, MD, FRCS (Urol); Adeboye O. Osunkoya, MD; Lance C. Pagliaro, MD; Michael A. Poch, MD; Praful Ravi, MBBChir; Wade J. Sexton, MD; Pranav Sharma, MD; Philippe E. Spiess, MD, MS, FRCS(C), FACS; Megan Suermann; Samer L. Traboulsi, MD; Alex J. Vanni, MD, FACS; Jared Wallen, MD; Nicholas A. Watkin, MA, MChir, FRCS (Urol); Lucas Wiegand, MD; Johannes Alfred Witjes, MD, PhD; Ding-Wei Ye, MD, PhD; Homayoun Zargar, MBChB, FRACS (Urol); Kamran Zargar-Shoshtari, MBChB, MD, FRACS; Yao Zhu, MD, PhD; Leonard N. Zinman, MD, FACS.

The planning committee, staff, authors and editors listed below have identified financial relationships or relationships to products or devices they or their spouse/life partner have with commercial interest related to the content of this CME activity:

Anna R. Giuliano, PhD has research support from, and is a consultant/advisor for, Merck & Co., Inc.

Shilpa Gupta, MD is a consultant/advisor for, and is on the speakers' bureau for, Genentech, Inc.

Guru Sonpavde, MD is a consultant/advisor for Merck & Co., Inc.; Genentech, Inc.; Sanofi; Pfizer Inc.; Novartis AG; Argos; Agensys, Inc.; and Bayer AG; and receives royalties/patents from UpToDate, Inc. and Clinical Care Options, LLC.

Samir S. Taneja, MD is a consultant/advisor for Bayer AG; Eigen Pharma LLC, GTx, Inc.; HealthTronics, Inc.; and Hitachi, Ltd.

UNAPPROVED/OFF-LABEL USE DISCLOSURE

The EOCME requires CME faculty to disclose to the participants:

1. When products or procedures being discussed are off-label, unlabelled, experimental, and/or investigational (not US Food and Drug Administration [FDA] approved); and
2. Any limitations on the information presented, such as data that are preliminary or that represent ongoing research, interim analyses, and/or unsupported opinions. Faculty may discuss information about pharmaceutical agents that is outside of FDA-approved labelling. This information is intended solely for CME and is not intended to promote off-label use of these medications. If you have any questions, contact the medical affairs department of the manufacturer for the most recent prescribing information.

TO ENROLL

To enroll in the *Urologic Clinics of North America* Continuing Medical Education program, call customer service at 1-800-654-2452 or sign up online at http://www.theclinics.com/home/cme. The CME program is available to subscribers for an additional annual fee of USD $270.

METHOD OF PARTICIPATION

In order to claim credit, participants must complete the following:

1. Complete enrolment as indicated above.
2. Read the activity.
3. Complete the CME Test and Evaluation. Participants must achieve a score of 70% on the test. All CME Tests and Evaluations must be completed online.

CME INQUIRIES/SPECIAL NEEDS

For all CME inquiries or special needs, please contact elsevierCME@elsevier.com.

Contributors

CONSULTING EDITOR

SAMIR S. TANEJA, MD
The James M. Neissa and Janet Riha Neissa
Professor of Urologic Oncology; Professor of
Urology and Radiology; Director, Division of
Urologic Oncology; Co-Director, Department
of Urology, Smilow Comprehensive Prostate
Cancer Center, NYU Langone Medical Center,
New York, New York

EDITOR

**PHILIPPE E. SPIESS, MD, MS, FRCS(C),
FACS**
Associate Member, Department of GU
Oncology; Associate Member, Department of
Tumor Biology, Moffitt Cancer Center;
Associate Professor, Department of Urology,
University of South Florida; Vice-Chair, NCCN
Bladder and Penile Cancer, Tampa, Florida

AUTHORS

JONATHAN BEILAN, MD
Department of Urology, University of South
Florida, Tampa, Florida

MICHAEL BICKELL, DO
Department of Urology, University of South
Florida, Tampa, Florida

MATT BROGGI, MSc
Medical Student, Emory University, Atlanta,
Georgia

RAFAEL CARRION, MD
Department of Urology, University of South
Florida, Tampa, Florida

JUANITA CROOK, MD, FRCPC
Professor of Radiation Oncology, University of
British Columbia, Center for the Southern
Interior, British Columbia Cancer Agency,
Kelowna, British Columbia, Canada

GREGORY J. DIORIO, DO
GU Oncology Fellow, Department of
Genitourinary Oncology, Moffitt Cancer
Center, Tampa, Florida

ANNA R. GIULIANO, PhD
Professor and Director, Center for Infection
Research in Cancer (CIRC), Moffitt Cancer
Center, Tampa, Florida

SHILPA GUPTA, MD
Department of Hematology, Oncology and
Transplantation, University of Minnesota,
Minneapolis, Minnesota

**PAUL K. HEGARTY, MB BCh BAO, Mch,
FRCSI, FRCS (Urol)**
Consultant Urological Surgeon; Department of
Urology, Mater Misericordiae University
Hospital and Mater Private, Dublin, Ireland

S. HORENBLAS, MD, PhD, FEBU
Chief; Professor, Department of Urology, Netherlands Cancer Institute, Amsterdam, The Netherlands

JONATHAN H. HUANG, MD
Urology Resident, Emory University, Atlanta, Georgia

WASSIM KASSOUF, MD, CM, FRCS(C)
Department of Urology, McGill University Health Centre, Montreal, Quebec, Canada

THARANI MAHESAN, MBBS, BSc, MRCS
Core Surgical Trainee; Penile Cancer Centre, St George's Healthcare NHS Trust, London, United Kingdom

VIRAJ A. MASTER, MD, PhD
Professor of Urology, Emory University, Atlanta, Georgia

S. MINHAS, MD, FRCS (Urol)
Consultant Urologist, University College Hospital, London, United Kingdom

ADEBOYE O. OSUNKOYA, MD
Professor of Pathology, Emory University, Atlanta, Georgia

LANCE C. PAGLIARO, MD
Professor of Oncology, Department of Oncology, Mayo Clinic, Rochester, Minnesota

MICHAEL A. POCH, MD
Assistant Member, Department of Genitourinary Oncology, Moffitt Cancer Center, Tampa, Florida

PRAFUL RAVI, MBBChir
Department of Internal Medicine, Mayo Clinic, Rochester, Minnesota

WADE J. SEXTON, MD
Senior Member and Professor, Department of Genitourinary Oncology, Moffitt Cancer Center, Tampa, Florida

PRANAV SHARMA, MD
GU Oncology Fellow, Department of Genitourinary Oncology, Moffitt Cancer Center, Tampa, Florida

GURU SONPAVDE, MD
Section of Medical Oncology, Department of Medicine, UAB Comprehensive Cancer Center, Birmingham, Alabama

PHILIPPE E. SPIESS, MD, MS, FRCS(C), FACS
Associate Member, Department of GU Oncology; Associate Member, Department of Tumor Biology, Moffitt Cancer Center; Associate Professor, Department of Urology, University of South Florida; Vice-Chair, NCCN Bladder and Penile Cancer, Tampa, Florida

SAMER L. TRABOULSI, MD
Department of Urology, McGill University Health Centre, Montreal, Quebec, Canada

ALEX J. VANNI, MD, FACS
Department of Urology, Lahey Hospital and Medical Center, Assistant Professor of Urology, Tufts University School of Medicine, Burlington, Massachusetts

JARED WALLEN, MD
Department of Urology, University of South Florida, Tampa, Florida

NICOLAS A. WATKIN, MA, MChir, FRCS (Urol)
Consultant Urological Surgeon, Head of Penile Cancer Centre, Penile Cancer Centre, St George's Healthcare NHS Trust, London, United Kingdom

LUCAS WIEGAND, MD
Department of Urology, University of South Florida, Tampa, Florida

JOHANNES ALFRED WITJES, MD, PhD
Department of Urology, Radboud University Nijmegen Medical Centre, Nijmegen, The Netherlands

DING-WEI YE, MD, PhD
Professor and Chairman, Department of Urology, Fudan University Shanghai Cancer Center; Department of Oncology, Shanghai Medical College, Fudan University, Shanghai, China

HOMAYOUN ZARGAR, MBChB, FRACS (Urol)
Australian Prostate Cancer Research Centre; Department of Urology, Royal Melbourne Hospital, Melbourne, Victoria, Australia

KAMRAN ZARGAR-SHOSHTARI, MBChB, MD, FRACS
Division of Urology, Department of Surgery, University of Auckland, Auckland, New Zealand

YAO ZHU, MD, PhD
Associate Professor, Department of Urology,
Fudan University Shanghai Cancer Center;
Department of Oncology, Shanghai Medical
College, Fudan University, Shanghai, China

LEONARD N. ZINMAN, MD, FACS
Department of Urology, Lahey Hospital and
Medical Center, Professor of Urology, Tufts
University School of Medicine, Burlington,
Massachusetts

Contents

Penile cancer is a rare and devastating disease, especially at advanced stages. The etiology of penile cancer is multifactorial with multiple established risk factors including infection with the human papillomavirus (HPV). Approximately 40% of penile cancers are attributable to HPV, although the literature describing HPV as a prognostic factor is mixed. The pathogenesis of HPV infection as well as vaccination practices may provide valuable therapeutic agents to treat this rare and difficult disease.

Penile-preserving surgery offers a revolutionary alternative to more traditional radical surgery. It offers better sexual, functional, and psychological results and evidence suggests it achieves this without sacrificing oncological outcomes. We examined the evolving nature of such surgeries, addressing controversies such as safe margins and survival outcomes and discussing more conventional techniques, including laser. At our UK center, we treat a high volume of penile cancer and here, based on such experience, we describe our glans resurfacing, glansectomy, and partial penectomy techniques; their application by disease stage; and the limitations of such surgeries.

Squamous cell cancer of the penis is a radiocurable malignancy all too often managed solely by partial or total penectomy. Effective management of the primary tumor while preserving penile morphology and function is a priority. External radiotherapy and brachytherapy have a role to play in the definitive management of the primary tumor. Surgical nodal staging remains a cornerstone of management because it is the strongest predictor of survival, and inguinal status determines pelvic management. Postoperative radiotherapy of the regional nodes for high-risk pathology is indicated. Chemoradiotherapy should be considered as neoadjuvant treatment for unresectable nodes or as definitive management.

> Penile cancer is a rare genitourinary malignancy. Lymph node involvement is the single most important factor determining survival in these patients, and those patients with occult disease are difficult to identify on conventional cross-sectional imaging. Until recently, lymph node sampling (eg, lymphadenectomy) has been the diagnostic modality of choice in the detection of micrometastasis. More recently, several novel molecular and minimally invasive diagnostic techniques have been developed, which have been demonstrated to decrease the false-negative and -positive results of conventional imaging and lymphadenectomy. This article focuses on the minimally invasive management of lymph nodes in men with penile cancer.

> Lymphadenectomy (LND) for locally advanced penile cancer is often necessary in patients with suspected disease within the inguinal or pelvic lymph nodes because the results of systemic therapy are somewhat marginal. It has utility in staging, disease prognosis, and treatment in certain men because early dissection of involved lymph nodes improves survival. Despite its mainstay in the management of this disease, inguinal and pelvic lymph node dissection can be associated with significant postoperative complications and patient morbidity. Recent refinements in surgical technique, however, and appropriate patient selection can minimize these risks and lead to better short-term and long-term outcomes.

> A multimodal approach to therapy is increasingly used in treating men with advanced penile cancer. Adjuvant chemotherapy improves outcomes in chemotherapy-naïve men with node-positive positive disease, and neoadjuvant chemotherapy can downstage bulky nodal disease sufficiently to permit surgery and has the potential to offer durable long-term survival. However, there remain several unanswered questions in this field, and international collaboration in the form of clinical trials is required to optimize treatment and improve survival in men with advanced penile cancer.

> Penile squamous cell carcinoma (PSCC) is a rare cancer, but is more common in developing countries. Locally advanced and metastatic PSCC is associated with significant morbidity and mortality, with the prognosis remaining extremely poor. The authors searched PubMed and published abstracts for metastatic PSCC studies to describe emerging therapies. Multimodality treatment using chemotherapy, radiation, and consolidative surgery are standard of care. Utilizing anti-EGFR therapies and novel immunotheraputic approaches may help improve outcomes in PSCC.

Primary urethral cancer is one of the rare urologic tumors. Distal urethral tumors are usually less advanced at diagnosis compared with proximal tumors and have a good prognosis if treated appropriately. Low-stage distal tumors can be managed successfully with a surgical approach in men or radiation therapy in women. There are no clear-cut indications for the choice of the most appropriate treatment modality. Organ-preserving modalities have shown effective and should be used whenever they do not compromise the oncological safety to decrease the physical and psychological trauma of dismemberment or loss of sexual/urinary function.

Primary urethral cancer (PUC) is a rare, but devastating genitourinary tumor that affects men and women. Although most PUC are localized, proximal PUC frequently presents with locally advanced disease, with 30% to 40% having lymph node metastasis. Single modality surgical or radiation therapy has dismal results. Multimodal therapy with cisplatin-based chemotherapy and consolidation surgery has greatly improved the local recurrence and overall survival rates for this aggressive disease. In locally advanced squamous cell carcinoma of the urethra, radiotherapy combined with radiosensitizing chemotherapy is an option for genital preservation. Prospective, multi-institutional studies are required to further define the optimal multidisciplinary treatment strategy for this destructive disease.

This article discusses the diagnostic and therapeutic options in the management of urethral cancer recurrence in patients treated with urethral sparing cystectomy as well as those who had urethral preservation following primary urethral carcinoma.

Occupational exposure has been causally linked to scrotal cancer. Primary preventative care and avoiding carcinogenic substances have decreased the incidence and changed the treatment of scrotal cancer. The current incidence of scrotal malignancy is approximately 1 per 1,000,000 male persons/year. The rarity of cases and of research impedes our understanding of the changing nature of scrotal cancer. This article summarizes the current knowledge, focusing mainly on pathogenesis and diagnostic evaluation, which may influence prevention and early recognition of the disease. We stratify scrotal cancer into common histologic subtypes: squamous cell carcinoma, extramammary Paget's disease, and basal cell carcinoma.

Primary scrotal cancer is a rare urologic malignancy with various histologic subtypes. Management and outcomes are not designed optimally. Surgical excision is the recommended treatment for localized scrotal cancer, with assessment of the margins for disease. Closure of the defect can be performed with primary closure, skin grafts, flaps, or by secondary intention. Analysis of outcomes suggests that high-risk scrotal cancer may have a worse prognosis compared with penile cancer, and low-risk scrotal cancer may have a comparable prognosis. Understanding techniques for management and survival outcomes can help the urologist determine the appropriate course of treatment and improve patient care.

UROLOGIC CLINICS OF NORTH AMERICA

THE CLINICS ARE AVAILABLE ONLINE!
Access your subscription at:
www.theclinics.com

Foreword
Penile, Urethral, and Scrotal Cancer

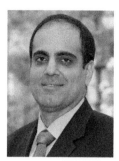

Samir S. Taneja, MD
Consulting Editor

Cancer of the male genitalia has historically been of great interest to urologists dating back to early history of the specialty. At the turn of the nineteenth century, Hugh Hampton Young changed the traditional approach to the disease following his observation that the lymphatic drainage of the penis was to the inguinal region and not through the scrotum, as originally thought. After this, the traditional approach of total penectomy, bilateral orchiectomy, and perineal urethrostomy was altered to preserve the scrotal contents and include the inguinal lymph nodes. Young also described preservation of the proximal penis to allow urination over the scrotum. Many of the principles described by Young in his 1931 publication persisted in the evolution of penile cancer surgery to modern day—surgical control of inguinal lymph nodes, wide margin local excision of the tumor, and penile preservation whenever possible. The recognition that penile cancer often has poor outcomes has prompted the use of multimodal approaches to maximize oncologic control.

Penile cancer has fallen out of the daily view of contemporary American urologists, largely owing to the broad implementation of circumcision in American culture, and the improved hygiene of the population that came with industrialization. In many parts of the country, penile cancer is of more historical significance than practical. This is even more true of scrotal cancer, which has become rare in the absence of known risk factors such as direct carcinogen exposure. Nonetheless, penile cancer, and to a lesser extent scrotal cancer, remains prevalent in many geographic regions and is frequently seen in urban areas where diverse ethnic and cultural populations may exist. Urethral cancer, often described as a rare manifestation within the broad context of urothelial cancer, is also something not frequently seen by the urologist in practice. In my view, it is critically important for urologists to be active in seeking out updates on the evolution of disease management for those diseases that they do not see on a daily basis. In this regard, an issue of *Urologic Clinics* devoted to penile, urethral, and scrotal cancers seemed timely and appropriate to me.

I would like to thank our guest editor, Dr Philippe E. Spiess, for his passionate devotion to the formulation and creation of this issue. He has crafted an extremely valuable resource for the practicing urologist, which includes all aspects of the management of these

Urol Clin N Am 43 (2016) xv–xvi
http://dx.doi.org/10.1016/j.ucl.2016.09.002
0094-0143/16/© 2016 Elsevier Inc. All rights reserved.

less-encountered malignancies, including nuances that one might not consider until they are actually confronted with the scenario in clinical practice. I am indebted to each of the authors for their wonderful contributions to the issue. It is my opinion that this issue will serve as the primary reference for American urologists, managing penile and urethral cancer, for years to come.

Samir S. Taneja, MD
Division of Urologic Oncology
Department of Urology
Smilow Comprehensive Prostate Cancer Center
NYU Langone Medical Center
150 East 32nd Street, Suite 200
New York, NY 10016, USA

E-mail address:
samir.taneja@nyumc.org

Preface
Penile, Urethral, and Scrotal Cancer

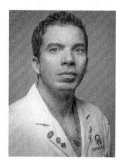

Philippe E. Spiess, MD, MS, FRCS(C), FACS
Editor

It is a distinct pleasure to serve as the guest editor for this issue of *Urologic Clinics* dedicated to the management of penile, urethral, and scrotal cancer. As a whole, these tumor entities are rare in their incidence and prevalence but in consequence impart significant heterogeneity in their diagnostic and therapeutic approaches. The present issue of *Urologic Clinics* encompasses contributions from thought leaders from around the world who share their expertise in the management of penile, urethral, and scrotal cancer while discussing the current standards of care using evidence-based treatment guidelines and providing insight as to emerging discoveries on these topics. A gathering of such leaders in these fields is invaluable to our readership as was so eloquently stated by the father of modern medicine, Sir William Osler (1849-1919), in that *"he who studies medicine without books sails an unchartered sea, but he who studies medicine without patients does not go to sea at all."*

The first articles of this issue are dedicated to discussing the fundamental role of the human papillomavirus in a significant subset of patients with penile cancer offering great potential for prevention using vaccination strategies among high-risk male populations. We subsequently discuss the role of penile-sparing surgical approaches in appropriately selected patients using a host of penile reconstructive techniques and principles. The role of radiation therapy as a treatment modality for both primary penile neoplasms and occult sites of disease is discussed by Dr Crook.

The selective role of radiation therapy in the neoadjuvant and adjuvant setting is touched upon as part of this discussion. The merit of minimally invasive diagnostic and surgical approaches in the evaluation of inguinal nodes is addressed by leading international experts in the field, Dr Horenblas and Dr Minhas. My group and I thereafter illustrate in our article some of the technical tips and tricks to inguinal lymph node surgery, which enhances oncologic outcomes while minimizing morbidity. One of the major advances in the field of penile cancer has been the adoption of a multimodal approach encompassing neoadjuvant systemic chemotherapy followed by surgical consolidative surgery among chemotherapy responders in patients with bulky (cN2/3) inguinal metastases secondary to penile cancer. This novel treatment paradigm was validated by a phase II clinical trial led by Dr Pagliaro, who has dedicated an article in the present issue in which he and his coauthor highlight the merits and curative potential of such an approach. We complete the present section by discussing emerging systemic therapies in the management of penile cancer, which encompasses very exciting advances in immunotherapeutics and targeted therapies specific to the epidermal growth factor receptor (among other) signal transduction pathways.

In the subsequent section, we highlight some of the suitable treatment strategies in the management of distal and noninvasive urethral tumors. We thereafter delve into the merits of multimodal

Urol Clin N Am 43 (2016) xvii–xviii
http://dx.doi.org/10.1016/j.ucl.2016.09.001
0094-0143/16/© 2016 Published by Elsevier Inc.

therapy in the management of proximal primary urethral tumors, which typically have an aggressive phenotype and have had traditionally disappointing oncologic outcomes with single-modality therapy, whether this be surgery, radiation, or systemic chemotherapy. We thereafter discuss the management of urethral recurrences of both urothelial and nonurothelial origin, which typically present late and portend an unfavorable prognosis.

In a section devoted to the management of primary scrotal cancer, colleagues from the Fudan University Shanghai Cancer Center highlight our current state of understanding with regard to the pathophysiology and diagnostic evaluation of primary scrotal cancer and its underlying preneoplastic condition. A detailed discussion of the surgical management of primary scrotal cancer follows. Last, a detailed overview of key surgical reconstructive techniques and approaches in the management of these penoscrotal neoplastic conditions is provided by colleagues from the University of South Florida.

I am confident this body of work will be greatly beneficial to colleagues and health care providers caring for patients facing such potentially debilitating diagnoses. In this regard, I would like to dedicate this issue to our patients and their families, whose heroism when faced with such adversity serves as an inspiration to us all. Thank you for the realization that good is not good enough and that until the complete eradication of cancer is accomplished, our mission is not achieved and we must quite simply do better.

Philippe E. Spiess, MD, MS, FRCS(C), FACS
Departments of GU Oncology and Tumor Biology
Moffitt Cancer Center
Department of Urology
University of South Florida
NCCN Bladder and Penile Cancer
12902 Magnolia Drive
Tampa, FL 33612, USA

E-mail address:
philippe.spiess@moffitt.org

The Role of Human Papilloma Virus in Penile Carcinogenesis and Preneoplastic Lesions
A Potential Target for Vaccination and Treatment Strategies

Gregory J. Diorio, DO[a],*, Anna R. Giuliano, PhD[b]

KEYWORDS

- HPV • Penile cancer • Penile –intraepithelial neoplasia (PeIN) • HPV vaccination • Targeted therapy

KEY POINTS

- Human papillomavirus (HPV) plays a crucial role in the development of penile cancer and its preneoplastic lesions.
- Understanding the pathogenesis of HPV in its relation to penile cancer may unlock new treatment pathways.
- HPV vaccination may reduce the incidence of HPV-related penile cancers and precancerous lesions.
- HPV-targeted therapies may play a role in treating local and advanced penile cancer.

INTRODUCTION

Although rare, penile cancer is a devastating disease, especially at advanced stages. The overall incidence in the United States and Western Europe is low, estimated to be 0.4% of all malignancies, although in parts of Africa, Asia, and South America it can reach an upwards of 10%.[1] The highest incidence occurs in men older than the age of 50 and is uncommon in younger men.[2] The etiology for penile cancer is multifactorial, with several factors identified, including phimosis, smoking, and chronic inflammatory states.[3] In certain penile tumors, there also seems to be a stepwise progression from precancerous external genital lesions to histologic carcinoma. Although the pathogenesis of penile cancer has yet to be fully elucidated, a clear association between human papillomavirus (HPV) infection and penile cancer has been established.[4] The advent and success of the quadrivalent vaccine against HPV has led to substantial decreases in HPV-associated infections and cancers in women, although studies have yet to demonstrate similar success in men specifically in relation to penile cancer and its precancerous lesions. The pathogenesis of HPV infection may provide valuable therapeutic agents to treat this rare and difficult

Disclosures: The author has nothing to disclose (G.J. Diorio); Receives research funding from Merck, Sharp & Dohme and serves as a consultant for the company related to HPV vaccines (A.R. Giuliano).
[a] Department of Genitourinary Oncology, Moffitt Cancer Center, 12902 USF Magnolia Drive, Tampa, FL 33612, USA; [b] Center for Infection Research in Cancer (CIRC), Moffitt Cancer Center, 12902 USF Magnolia Drive, MRC-CANCONT, Tampa, FL 33612, USA
* Corresponding author.
E-mail address: gregory.diorio@moffitt.org

disease. In this review, we describe the role of HPV in penile cancer and its associated preneoplastic lesions.

HUMAN PAPILLOMAVIRUS PATHOGENESIS AND PENILE CANCER

HPV is a nonenveloped DNA virus that exists in the highly mitotic keratinocytes and mucous membranes. Infection by viral proteins causes loss of regulation of the cell cycle controlling proliferation and apoptosis, leading to dysplasia and, potentially, carcinogenesis.[5] The vast majority of infections are cleared by the host's immune system and infections remain asymptomatic and self-limiting.[5] HPV has been implicated in several malignancies, including cervical, oropharynx, anal, and penile. Approximately 500,000 new cancer diagnoses will be directly attributed to HPV infection each year.[6] The majority of these cases will be cervical cancer, where HPV DNA is detected in nearly 100% of tumor specimens. In contrast, approximately 40% of penile cancers are thought to be attributed to HPV infection.[7]

Penile cancer predominantly contains squamous cell histology, although several subtypes exist including basaloid, warty, keratinizing, and verrucous. Basaloid and warty histologies have been associated with HPV infection, whereas the remaining subtypes rarely contain HPV DNA.[8] A study by Rubin and colleagues[4] examined the presence of HPV DNA in penile carcinoma subtypes, precancerous lesions, and condyloma using an HPV polymerase chain reaction assay and genotyping line probe assay. HPV DNA was found in 42% of penile carcinoma cases, 90% of dysplasias, and 100% of condylomas. Keratinizing squamous cell carcinoma and verrucous subtypes showed the lowest percentage of HPV DNA at 34.9% and 33.3%, respectively, whereas basaloid and warty types had 80% and 100%.

Two pathophysiologic mechanisms have been proposed to contribute to the development of penile cancer and its associated premalignant lesions, the first related to proinflammatory conditions such as chronic balanitis, phimosis, and lichen sclerosis/balanitis xerotica obliterans and the second owing to HPV infection. Several hundred genotypes of the HPV virus have been described affecting both cutaneous and mucosal sites and generally classified into "low risk" and "high risk" according to their association with cervical malignancy. Although 13 to 15 HPV types are described as high risk for cervical cancer, only 1 HPV type, HPV-16, is considered a cause of penile cancer. HPV-6 and HPV-11 have been implicated in benign lesions such as condyloma acuminate

and are considered low risk for malignant transformation. In cervical cancers, high-risk HPV-16 has been implicated in approximately 50% of cases and HPV-18 another 15% to 20%.[9] Similarly, studies in penile cancer have demonstrated the presence of high-risk HPV-16 and HPV-18 in approximately 70% of penile cancers, with HPV-16 being the predominant subtype.[10]

It remains unclear whether HPV-related penile cancers have an improved survival profile compared with cancers unrelated to HPV infection. Bezerra and colleagues[11] demonstrated that, in 82 patients with penile cancer, 30.5% of tumors contained HPV DNA with HPV-16 the most prevalent type at 52%. No difference was seen between HPV negative and positive patients in terms of lymph node metastasis ($P = .386$) and the 10-year survival rate (68.4% vs 69.1%; $P = .83$). A similar study by Wiener and colleagues[12] demonstrated no association between tumor HPV status with risk of nodal metastasis or survival. In contrast, Lont and colleagues[13] examined HPV status as a prognostic indicator in 171 patients with penile cancer. High-risk HPV DNA was detected in 29% of tumors with 76% containing HPV-16. The presence of high-risk HPV was associated with an improved 5-year disease-specific survival (78% vs 93%; $P = .03$) and was an independent predictor of disease specific mortality in multivariate analysis (hazard ratio, 0.14; 95% CI, 0.03–0.63; $P = .01$). Study design, sample size, and sampling methods for HPV DNA likely contribute to the conflicting results and routine testing, especially because HPV DNA testing of penile squamous cell carcinoma tumors has yet to be adopted universally.

HUMAN PAPILLOMAVIRUS PREVALENCE AND PENILE CANCER

In contrast with cervical cancer, where nearly 100% of tumor cells contain HPV DNA, the prevalence of HPV DNA in penile cancer varies throughout the literature. Alemany and colleagues[14] described the prevalence of HPV in penile cancer tumor and precancerous lesions in a large international study from 25 countries. A total of 85 precancerous lesions and 1010 penile cancers were diagnosed. HPV DNA was detected in 33.1% of penile tumors and 87.1% of precancerous lesions. Recent studies from national registries in Denmark have suggested that the overall incidence of penile cancer may be increasing. The incidence of penile cancer increased 1.0 to 1.3 per 100,000 men from 1978 to 2008 for and estimated annual percent change of 0.8% (95% CI, 0.17–1.37). Similarly, the incidence of precancerous lesions increased from 1998 to 2008 from 0.5 to 0.9 per 100,000 men representing an annual percent change of 7.1% (95% CI, 3.30–11.05). The authors conclude that a high prevalence of HPV (33%–65%) as well as low circumcision rates may be the causative factors.[15]

HPV prevalence seems to be increasing worldwide, although variations in the literature may be owing to the differences in sampling methods, molecular testing, and populations studied.[6] The global prevalence of HPV infection in women has been estimated to be 11% to 12% with the highest prevalence observed in sub-Saharan Africa, Eastern Europe, and Latin America. The prevalence of HPV in men varies with most studies reporting estimates of greater than 20%, with a lower prevalence in circumcised men versus uncircumcised men.[16,17] Most HPV infections do not result in pathogenic external lesions and are immunologically cleared by 12 months, with 1 study of men in the United States reporting a median clearance time of 5.9 months.[18] A study examining the prevalence of HPV in men and boys from prepuce samples in the absence of external lesions demonstrated that high-risk HPV subtypes were found in 45.5% of children (ages 0–10 years), 60.6% of adolescents (11–20 years), and 58.3% in adults (>20 years). The greatest prevalence of high-risk HPV at 59.8% was reported in age groups with the highest estimated rates of sexual activity (>14 years). These results support the concept that HPV is very common in males owing to the consistent prevalence of HPV in men across age groups and reinforces the usefulness of vaccination protocols in boys and young adults.[19]

HUMAN PAPILLOMAVIRUS AND PRENEOPLASTIC LESIONS

HPV infection is associated with 2 types of external genital lesions: condyloma acuminate (genital warts) and precancerous external genital lesions. The histologic precancerous lesions associated with squamous cell carcinomas of the penis have been termed penile intraepithelial neoplasia (PeIN). PeIN lesions themselves can have wide range of morphology and multiple classifications have been proposed.[20,21] As defined by Cubilla and colleagues,[21] PeIN can be classified into differentiated and undifferentiated categories. Differentiated PeIN is generally associated with conditions of chronic inflammation such as lichen sclerosis and is thought to progress to well-differentiated and keratinized squamous cell carcinoma.[20,22] Undifferentiated PeIN is considered to be a premalignant lesion for HPV-associated penile cancer

subtypes basaloid and warty squamous cell carcinoma.[23] Approximately 60% to 100% of PeIN lesions contain HPV DNA with the vast majority containing HPV-16.[24] In a report from the HPV in Men international study, 14 patients developed external genital lesions diagnosed as PeIN. In 85.7%, there was more than 1 type of high risk HPV and 57.1% contained HPV-16.[25] In a follow-up study of this large international collaboration of more than 1700 HPV- positive men sampled, 9 developed external genital lesion classified as PeIN. Again the vast majority of PeIN lesions contained the HPV-16 subtype. During the first 12 months of follow-up, 0.5% of men with a genital HPV-16 infection developed an HPV-16–positive PeIN. Again, the small sample size and rarity of PeIN lesions in general prevent a robust analysis from being performed.[26] The authors emphasize that of all the lesions detected all could be prevented with vaccine administration.

HUMAN PAPILLOMAVIRUS VACCINATION STRATEGIES IN MEN

HPV infects the genital squamous epithelium of men and women with similar incidence, although women have a greater proportion of seropositivity and higher antibody levels. Men seem to have a less robust immune response, which may be responsible for the higher prevalence of HPV infection seen in males and consistency of distribution across age groups.[27] This is in contrast with women, where the greatest prevalence is seen is women 18 to 24 years old and then decreases through middle age.[28]

In the only phase III vaccine trial to date that evaluated HPV vaccine efficacy against infection and clinical disease, the quadrivalent HPV vaccine directed against HPV types 6, 11, 16, and 18 was shown to be highly efficacious. Giuliano and colleagues[27] described the use of the vaccine in males ages 16 to 26 with primary endpoints being HPV vaccine type related external genital lesions (condyloma acuminate, penile/perianal/perianal intraepithelial neoplasia, and associated cancers) and persistent HPV-6, -11, -16, or -18 genital infections. The results demonstrated an efficacy of 90.4% (95% CI, 45.8–98.1) against lesions related to HPV-6, -11, -16, or -18 in the per protocol population. Efficacy in terms of prevention of persistent infection to HPV-6, -11, -16, or -18 was 85.6% (97.5% CI, 73.4–92.9). A small percentage of patients in the study group had lesions classified as PeIN and no patients in either group had associated malignancy. On the basis of these data, the US Food and Drug Administration approved the vaccine for the prevention of genital warts in males ages 9 to 26 in 2009 and the Advisory Committee on Immunization Practices of the Centers for Disease Control and Prevention recommended routine vaccination of males as well as females in 2011. However, because too few PeIN lesions (3 cases in the placebo arm only) were accrued, there was insufficient information to allow conclusions related to PeIN and penile cancer prevention. Thus, there is no recommendation for vaccine use for the prevention of penile precancerous lesions and squamous cell carcinoma of the penis. Direct correlations for the reduction of HPV associated PeIN and penile cancer warrant further investigation.

Despite the approval and availability of the HPV vaccine for males internationally, there remains a widespread lack of knowledge about HPV-associated diseases and the need for vaccination programs directed at males. In a European study of 900 patients seen for urologic issues, only 51% percent reported knowledge of HPV.[29] Of those who were aware of HPV, only 58.5% were aware that HPV infection is associated with penile cancer and only 36.5% were aware of an available vaccine to prevent these infections. Thus, bridging the gap in public knowledge of HPV acquisition and its association with genitourinary cancers will pave the way for preventative strategies against infection in the future and in turn encourage further education and standardized vaccination practices.

TARGETED THERAPIES IN HUMAN PAPILLOMAVIRUS–ASSOCIATED MALIGNANCY

The oncogenic effects of the high-risk HPV-16 and HPV-18 are mediated through 3 distinct oncogenes: E5, E6, and E7. The activation of E5 is not necessarily required for malignant progression, although it may contribute to carcinogenesis by influencing viral uptake into host target cells and subsequent development of dysplasia associated with premalignant lesions. The E5 oncogene produces a transmembrane protein that regulates activation of tyrosine receptor kinase epidermal growth factor receptor (EGFR). EGFR upregulation causes a reduction in E-cadherin expression that, together with an associated increase in MMP-9, decreases cell-to cell adhesion.[30] Pharmacologic blockade of EGFR has been shown to have therapeutic benefits in patients with squamous cell carcinomas of the head and neck as well as penile carcinoma.[30] Necchi and colleagues[31] described a case report of a patient with recurrent metastatic squamous cell carcinoma of the penis treated with anti-EGFR agent panitumumab with a complete and durable clinical response. Similarly, Carthon

and colleagues[32] published a retrospective case series of 24 patients with metastatic disease treated with anti-EGFR–targeted agents cetuximab (67%), erlotinib, and gefitnib in conjunction with convention chemotherapy. The median overall survival for these patients was encouraging at 29.6 weeks, despite the vast majority of patients having recurrent or progressive disease. With these promising results, several ongoing clinical trials are exploring the role of EGFR-targeted therapies in patients with penile cancer. The role HPV infection in conjunction with EGFR status may be a crucial factor for predicting treatment response in the future, although further prospective trials are warranted.

Unlike E5, the E6 and E7 oncogenes are necessary for the malignant transformation and maintenance of the malignant phenotype in HPV-associated malignancy. E6 and E7 both function through inhibition of 2 vital tumor suppressor genes: p53 and retinoblastoma tumor-suppressor protein (Rb) (**Fig. 1**). The increased degradation of p53 and Rb allows the promotion of viral replication and ultimately disrupts the host's normal cell cycle leading to malignant transformation. E6 and E7 also contribute to carcinogenesis by promoting mutations in genes central to mitosis. The oncogenes disrupt centrosome synthesis, resulting in the formation of multipolar mitosis that has been characterized as a hallmark feature of both HPV-induced premalignant lesions and malignant tumors. Ultimately, a higher mutation rate occurs and transformed cells are permitted to propagate, whereas they would normally be kept in check by tumor suppressors and cell cycle check points.

Because both oncogenes E6 and E7 play a vital part in the role of HPV in carcinogenesis, they also serve as potential therapeutic targets. Several strategies gave been proposed to disrupt the E6/E7 pathway from direct inhibition of RNA expression to targeting downstream targets of the oncogenes. Although ideal for therapeutic intervention, the success at targeting the HPV genome in HPV-related cancers has been limited.[33,34]

With the advent of HPV vaccination recommendations, the prevalence of HPV will ultimately decrease, as will HPV-associated malignancies. However, multiple generations of men who are outside the recommended age of vaccination remains at risk for PeIN and penile cancer. Until there is broad vaccine dissemination to age eligible males, the decrease in penile cancer incidence will not be seen, likely for decades. The time frame for the vaccine reduction of penile cancer will also be prolonged by inconsistent vaccine practices.

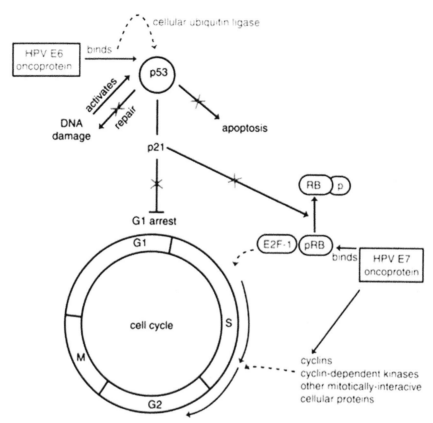

Fig. 1. Pathogenesis of human papillomavirus (HPV). (*From* Burd EM. Human papillomavirus and cervical cancer. Clin Microbiol Rev 2003;16(1):5; with permission.)

Therapeutic vaccine strategies targeting the E6 and E7 oncogenes have been proposed with some success. The HPV-16 E6/E7 peptide vaccine has shown to invoke a robust host immune response of CD4 and CD8 T cells in a small study of patients with cervical cancer.[34] A similar trial in patients with HPV-16–positive vulvar cancer demonstrated promising clinical and immunologic responses.[35] Other strategies using nonpeptide mechanisms of introducing HPV DNA to evoke an immune response have been described including the use of bacterial strains and adenovirus strains as vector mechanisms. A combined therapeutic and prophylactic vaccine to HPV-16 and E7 genes has been developed, although clinical studies demonstrated limited therapeutic efficacy in patients with precursor cervical intraepithelial lesions.[36] No therapeutic vaccine studies have been performed in patients with penile cancer to date.

Perhaps the most promising work with targeting HPV-associated malignancy has been seen with adoptive T-cell therapy. Adoptive T-cell therapy involves harvesting patient-specific T cells from primary tumor or metastatic sites and establishing a T-cell culture. The T-cell cultures from HPV-positive cancers are then selected for reactivity to HPV-16, HPV-18, and to the oncoproteins E6 and E7 and expanded. These HPV-targeted tumor-infiltrating lymphocytes are then able to be infused to the donor patients in hope of inducing enough of an immune response for tumor destruction.

Stevanovic and colleagues[37] infused 9 patients with metastatic cervical cancer with an autologous HPV tumor-infiltrating lymphocytes. Three patients experienced a clinical response with 2 patients achieving a prolonged complete regression of metastatic disease at a follow-up of 22 and 15 months. Clinical response was associated with HPV reactivity of the T-cell infusion product ($P = .02$) and the frequency of HPV reactive T cells in the peripheral blood 1 month after treatment ($P = .02$).[37] The downside to these exciting therapies is the cost and time needed to produce a viable and biologically active product. An incubation period of approximately 6 weeks is needed to culture the reactive T cells, a time period which that may have serious implications for patients with metastatic disease who are refractory to conventional therapy. The expensive and time-consuming process may also not yield enough active cells for infusion. In conjunction, the patients also need preinfusion treatment with lymphocyte-depleting chemotherapy followed by cytokine induction, a process that is not without significant morbidity. Although no studies involving HPV-targeted agents have been published in HPV-positive penile cancer to date, these findings are promising; future directions in the management of advanced penile cancer and several trials are ongoing to examine adoptive T-cell therapy in this difficult-to-treat population.

SUMMARY

HPV is a common sexually transmitted infection that has several implications for the development of penile cancer and its precancerous lesions. The true prognostic implications of HPV-associated penile cancer have yet to be elucidated fully, although studies in other squamous cell carcinomas, specifically of the head and neck, have shown promising results. Certainly with the development of the quadrivalent HPV vaccine and the adoption of universal vaccination practices, the incidence of HPV-associated cancers and precancerous lesions will decrease, especially in those countries with gender-neutral HPV vaccine policies. In practice, widespread vaccination will also help to curb the increasing cost of treating and managing these difficult conditions. Although the development of a therapeutic vaccine for high-risk HPV subtypes has been disappointing further research is ongoing and may be a cost-effective and practical strategy.

As the molecular pathways of HPV DNA pathogenesis are further unraveled, potential therapeutic targets have been discovered that may have serious implications for the treatment of this disease in advanced stages. Although the prognosis for patients with advanced penile cancer is poor, future studies combining HPV status with conventional systemic treatments need to be explored. The addition of novel targeted therapies may be the key to providing a practical and durable survival benefit in this difficult population.

REFERENCES

1. Bleeker MC, Heideman DA, Snijders PJ, et al. Penile cancer: epidemiology, pathogenesis and prevention. World J Urol 2009;27:141–50.
2. Pizzocaro G, Algaba F, Horenblas S, et al. EAU penile cancer guidelines 2009. Eur Urol 2010;57: 1002–12.
3. Daling JR, Madeleine MM, Johnson LG, et al. Penile cancer: importance of circumcision, human papillomavirus and smoking in in situ and invasive disease. Int J Cancer 2005;116:606–16.
4. Rubin MA, Kleter B, Zhou M, et al. Detection and typing of human papillomavirus DNA in penile carcinoma: evidence for multiple independent pathways of penile carcinogenesis. Am J Pathol 2001;159: 1211–8.
5. Flaherty A, Kim T, Giuliano A, et al. Implications for human papillomavirus in penile cancer. Urol Oncol 2014;32:53.e1-8.
6. Forman D, de Martel C, Lacey CJ, et al. Global burden of human papillomavirus and related diseases. Vaccine 2012;30(Suppl 5):F12–23.
7. IARC Working Group on the Evaluation of Carcinogenic Risks to Humans. Human papillomaviruses. IARC Monogr Eval Carcinog Risks Hum 2007;90: 1–636.
8. Kalantari M, Villa LL, Calleja-Macias IE, et al. Human papillomavirus-16 and -18 in penile carcinomas: DNA methylation, chromosomal recombination and genomic variation. Int J Cancer 2008;123:1832–40.
9. Munoz N, Bosch FX, de Sanjose S, et al. Epidemiologic classification of human papillomavirus types associated with cervical cancer. N Engl J Med 2003;348:518–27.
10. Carter JJ, Madeleine MM, Shera K, et al. Human papillomavirus 16 and 18 L1 serology compared across anogenital cancer sites. Cancer Res 2001; 61:1934–40.
11. Bezerra AL, Lopes A, Santiago GH, et al. Human papillomavirus as a prognostic factor in carcinoma of the penis: analysis of 82 patients treated with amputation and bilateral lymphadenectomy. Cancer 2001;91:2315–21.
12. Wiener JS, Effert PJ, Humphrey PA, et al. Prevalence of human papillomavirus types 16 and 18 in squamous-cell carcinoma of the penis: a retrospective analysis of primary and metastatic lesions by differential polymerase chain reaction. Int J Cancer 1992;50:694–701.
13. Lont AP, Kroon BK, Horenblas S, et al. Presence of high-risk human papillomavirus DNA in penile carcinoma predicts favorable outcome in survival. Int J Cancer 2006;119:1078–81.
14. Alemany L, Cubilla A, Halec G, et al. Role of Human Papillomavirus in Penile Carcinomas Worldwide. Eur Urol 2016;69(5):953–61.
15. Baldur-Felskov B, Hannibal CG, Munk C, et al. Increased incidence of penile cancer and high-grade penile intraepithelial neoplasia in Denmark 1978-2008: a nationwide population-based study. Cancer Causes Control 2012;23:273–80.
16. Dunne EF, Nielson CM, Stone KM, et al. Prevalence of HPV infection among men: A systematic review of the literature. J Infect Dis 2006;194:1044–57.

17. Castellsague X, Bosch FX, Munoz N, et al. Male circumcision, penile human papillomavirus infection, and cervical cancer in female partners. N Engl J Med 2002;346:1105–12.

18. Lu B, Wu Y, Nielson CM, et al. Factors associated with acquisition and clearance of human papillomavirus infection in a cohort of US men: a prospective study. J Infect Dis 2009;199:362–71.

19. Klinglmair G, Pichler R, Zelger B, et al. Prevalence of the human papillomavirus (HPV) expression of the inner prepuce in asymptomatic boys and men. World J Urol 2013;31:1389–94.

20. Velazquez EF, Chaux A, Cubilla AL. Histologic classification of penile intraepithelial neoplasia. Semin Diagn Pathol 2012;29:96–102.

21. Cubilla AL, Velazquez EF, Young RH. Epithelial lesions associated with invasive penile squamous cell carcinoma: a pathologic study of 288 cases. Int J Surg Pathol 2004;12:351–64.

22. Chaux A, Pfannl R, Lloveras B, et al. Distinctive association of p16INK4a overexpression with penile intraepithelial neoplasia depicting warty and/or basaloid features: a study of 141 cases evaluating a new nomenclature. Am J Surg Pathol 2010;34:385–92.

23. Gregoire L, Cubilla AL, Reuter VE, et al. Preferential association of human papillomavirus with high-grade histologic variants of penile-invasive squamous cell carcinoma. J Natl Cancer Inst 1995;87:1705–9.

24. Aynaud O, Ionesco M, Barrasso R. Penile intraepithelial neoplasia. Specific clinical features correlate with histologic and virologic findings. Cancer 1994;74:1762–7.

25. Ingles DJ, Pierce Campbell CM, Messina JA, et al. Human papillomavirus virus (HPV) genotype- and age-specific analyses of external genital lesions among men in the HPV Infection in Men (HIM) Study. J Infect Dis 2015;211:1060–7.

26. Sudenga SL, Ingles DJ, Pierce Campbell CM, et al. Genital human papillomavirus infection progression to external genital lesions: the HIM study. Eur Urol 2016;69:166–73.

27. Giuliano AR, Palefsky JM, Goldstone S, et al. Efficacy of quadrivalent HPV vaccine against HPV Infection and disease in males. N Engl J Med 2011;364:401–11.

28. Burchell AN, Winer RL, de Sanjose S, et al. Chapter 6: epidemiology and transmission dynamics of genital HPV infection. Vaccine 2006;24(Suppl 3):S3/52-61.

29. Capogrosso P, Ventimiglia E, Matloob R, et al. Awareness and knowledge of human papillomavirus-related diseases are still dramatically insufficient in the era of high-coverage vaccination programs. World J Urol 2015;33:873–80.

30. Agarwal G, Gupta S, Spiess PE. Novel targeted therapies for the treatment of penile cancer. Expert Opin Drug Discov 2014;9:959–68.

31. Necchi A, Nicolai N, Colecchia M, et al. Proof of activity of anti-epidermal growth factor receptor-targeted therapy for relapsed squamous cell carcinoma of the penis. J Clin Oncol 2011;29:e650–2.

32. Carthon BC, Ng CS, Pettaway CA, et al. Epidermal growth factor receptor-targeted therapy in locally advanced or metastatic squamous cell carcinoma of the penis. BJU Int 2014;113:871–7.

33. Trimble CL, Frazer IH. Development of therapeutic HPV vaccines. Lancet Oncol 2009;10:975–80.

34. Trimble CL, Morrow MP, Kraynyak KA, et al. Safety, efficacy, and immunogenicity of VGX-3100, a therapeutic synthetic DNA vaccine targeting human papillomavirus 16 and 18 E6 and E7 proteins for cervical intraepithelial neoplasia 2/3: a randomised, double-blind, placebo-controlled phase 2b trial. Lancet 2015;386:2078–88.

35. Davidson EJ, Boswell CM, Sehr P, et al. Immunological and clinical responses in women with vulval intraepithelial neoplasia vaccinated with a vaccinia virus encoding human papillomavirus 16/18 oncoproteins. Cancer Res 2003;63:6032–41.

36. Kaufmann AM, Nieland JD, Jochmus I, et al. Vaccination trial with HPV16 L1E7 chimeric virus-like particles in women suffering from high grade cervical intraepithelial neoplasia (CIN 2/3). Int J Cancer 2007;121:2794–800.

37. Stevanovic S, Draper LM, Langhan MM, et al. Complete regression of metastatic cervical cancer after treatment with human papillomavirus-targeted tumor-infiltrating T cells. J Clin Oncol 2015;33:1543–50.

Advances in Penile-Preserving Surgical Approaches in the Management of Penile Tumors

Tharani Mahesan, MBBS, BSc, MRCS[a],
Paul K. Hegarty, MB BCh BAO, Mch, FRCSI, FRCS (Urol)[b],
Nicolas A. Watkin, MA, MChir, FRCS (Urol)[a],*

KEYWORDS

- Penile-preserving surgery • Glansectomy • Penectomy • Glans resurfacing • Laser

KEY POINTS

- Penile-preserving surgery offers good functional and sexual results without sacrificing oncological outcomes.
- In accordance to European Association of Urology guidelines, safe margins in penile-preserving surgery are set at 5 mm but studies suggest they can be as little as 1 mm without sacrificing on oncological outcomes.
- When compared with more radical surgical techniques, penile-preserving surgery does not reduce survival but can lead to a higher rate of local recurrence.

The incidence of penile cancer is increasing and its treatment evolving. Traditional radical surgery, although admittedly often overtreatment of the primary lesion, had offered excellent oncological outcomes but with high physical and psychosexual morbidity. Instead, urologists are increasingly performing penile-preserving surgeries with the aim of achieving good oncological control with minimal functional and anatomic disruption.[1]

The aim of this article was to provide a thorough and relevant update on the advancements of penile-preserving surgical techniques in high-volume UK centers.

WHAT IS AN ONCOLOGICALLY SAFE MARGIN?

The turning point for penile-preserving surgeries came in 2005 with the introduction of new European Association of Urology guidelines.[2] Historically, it was believed that adequate clearance required a 2-cm tumor-free margin; however, the new guidelines set this at just 5 mm, reflecting a new body of evidence that questioned that belief.

In 2000, Agrawal and colleagues[3] reviewed 64 partial and total penectomy specimens with a view to determining the microscopic spread of the tumor beyond macroscopic margins. They concluded that 81% did not extend beyond visible tumor margins and of those that did, only 25% (3/64) extended more than 5 mm from the margin. Minhas and colleagues[4] performed a similar study, this time assessing penile-preserving techniques. They concluded that despite 92% of patients having a less than 20-mm margin (48% of which was <10 mm), only 3 (6%) patients had positive margins and only 2 (4%) developed local tumor recurrence within an average of 26 months [39]. Both

Conflict of Interest: No potential conflicts of interest. No financial support.
[a] Department of Urology, Penile Cancer Centre, St George's Healthcare NHS Trust, Blackshaw road, London SW17 0QT, UK; [b] Department of Urology, Mater Misericordiae University Hospital and Mater Private, Eccles Street, Dublin 7, Ireland
* Corresponding author.
E-mail address: nick.watkin@stgeorges.nhs.uk

Urol Clin N Am 43 (2016) 427–434
http://dx.doi.org/10.1016/j.ucl.2016.06.004

studies adding support to the hypothesis that excision margins of less than 10 mm had no bearing on recurrence.[5]

More recently, a study of 332 patients demonstrated no significant relationship between margins of less than 5 mm and local recurrence. A margin of less than 1 mm, however, was associated with a significantly increased risk. Other factors influencing local recurrence included lympho-vascular invasion and cavernosal involvement. The investigators concluded that a deep clear tumor-free margin of 1 mm or more was sufficient in penile-preserving surgery (D Sri, A Sujenthiran, W Lam, C Corbishley, BE Ayres, N Watkin. The significance of close surgical margins in organ sparing surgery for penile squamous cell cancer. Accepted for presentation BAUS, 2016, personal communication).

With reduced tumor-free margins, positive margins are undoubtedly a risk. Those with positive margins require either early re-resection or active surveillance. An as-yet unpublished study of 42 patients with positive margins at our regional penile cancer center showed that only 6 had residual disease. They recommended that patients with contiguous deep margin, delayed graft healing, or extensive positive margins may benefit from early surgical intervention. Others should be closely monitored with a specialist clinic, as studies have demonstrated that local recurrence does not compromise long-term survival because most recurrences are still surgically salvageable.[4,6–9]

WHAT SURGICAL OPTIONS ARE AVAILABLE BY DISEASE STAGE?

The stage and location of the primary lesion need to be considered when selecting the most appropriate technique. The patient's age and comorbidities, and the impact of any potential loss of penile length also should be taken into account.

The management of the premalignant or malignant penile lesion is not limited to surgery. For those with proven noninvasive disease, isolated to the distal portion of the penis, topical therapies including chemo, immune, and photodynamic therapies offer viable alternatives. These are often offered with circumcision for ease of follow-up and to reduce infection risk.

Traditionally, the decision on whether to pursue topical chemotherapy or laser treatments is determined by staging from incisional biopsies. However, increasing evidence suggests that such biopsies may be understaging the extent of disease invasion, resulting in the use of topical treatment that do not address invasive components. This may explain the high recurrence rates seen with topical treatments and lasers. This supports the use of penile-preserving surgery as primary treatment, allowing to more accurately stage the tumor and to avoid the severe consequences that could occur as a result of underestimating the nature the disease.[8,10,11]

For Lesions Confined to the Prepuce: Circumcision

The role of circumcision in the management of penile cancer is multifaceted. From a therapeutic standpoint, it is suitable for any lesion confined solely to the prepuce. It can play a preventive role in those with superficial glanular lesions (Tis), as its removal results in the loss of a human papillomavirus (HPV)-favorable micro-environment that, with time, could result in chronic inflammation and invasive disease. Finally, it facilitates clinical examination, which is vital for long-term follow-up.

When performing a circumcision, the surgeon should ensure adequate tumor-free margin and examine the glans for disease. Surgeons may apply acetic acid to guide excision margins; however, concerns about sensitivity and false-positive staining persist, in particular with regard to HPV detection.[12–14]

For Glanular Lesions up to T1a

Glans resurfacing

Total glans resurfacing was first described by Depasquale and colleagues[15] for the treatment of balanitis xerotica obliterans. Since being adapted for Tis, it has become the gold standard surgical treatment for glanular lesions up to T1a; however, partial glans resurfacing may be offered in the absence of multifocal tumor, if glanular involvement is below 50% and only for tumors up to Ta.

Patients should be administered preoperative antibiotics on induction of their general anesthetic, and a penile tourniquet used for control of hemostasis. In total glans resurfacing, all epithelium and subepithelium of the glans are marked and excised leaving only a perimeatal and circumcoronal margin. This is undertaken in quadrants starting from the meatus to the coronal sulcus for each quadrant. Frozen specimens of deep spongiosal tissue may be taken from each quadrant to exclude invasion.

The split-thickness grafts, harvested from thigh, should include an air dermatome and be between 0.008 and 0.016 in thickness. The graft should be sutured and quilted with 5 to 0 interrupted vicryl sutures and dressed with a soft paraffin gauze followed by a foam dressing. A catheter should be placed to keep the wound clean and dry and the patient is then placed on 48-hour strict bed rest.

The dressing and catheter should be removed on the fifth day before discharge, with a plan for wound review after 1 week.

Partial glans resurfacing applies the same principles as total glans resurfacing but has the added benefit of conserving normal glans skin. It therefore offers preservation of normal glanular sensation and better cosmesis, although with this, carries a high risk of positive surgical margins.[10] Low rates of recurrence, however, are reported, with a study of 36 patients with T disease citing a 6% recurrence rate.[16] Evidence suggests that, where possible, partial glans resurfacing may be more attractive to young, sexually active men, although all should be counseled that further surgical intervention may be required, which may be in the form of total glans resurfacing or glansectomy.

Glans resurfacing, like wide local excision (WLE; discussed later in this article) is most appropriate in those with low-grade disease in the absence of lymphovascular invasion. An emphasis should be placed on regular self-examination and patients should be carefully selected in an attempt to ensure compliance with follow-up.

Outcome reporting for glans resurfacing is largely positive, reporting good functional and cosmetic results (**Table 1**). Shabbir and colleagues[10] reported 96% total graft uptake in their study of 25 patients, with Hadway and colleagues[11] reporting 100% uptake in theirs. Neither study reported any postoperative complications and both the investigators and Hakansson and colleagues[17] denied recurrence (up to 30 months in the case of Shabbir and colleagues[10]) after total glans resurfacing. Sexual function was preserved, with one study noting that WLE led to better sexual outcomes when compared with glansectomy.[11] Despite clear benefits to glans resurfacing, positive margins persist as a challenge, with 48% of a mixed partial and total glans resurfacing cohort affected and 28% requiring further surgery most often in the form of total or partial glansectomy[10] (**Figs. 1–4**).

Laser therapy

Laser therapy is best suited for Tis but has been used up to T2 lesions. It exists in 2 main forms: the more deeply penetrating coagulative laser (Nd:YAG; 3–5-mm depth) and vaporizing lasers (carbon dioxide or holmium), which have a much shorter depth of penetration (2.0–2.5 mm). The carbon dioxide laser offers a "scalpel" technique allowing for histologic analysis of excised tissue. Nd:YAG lasers, however, cause tissue coagulation of the base of the tumor. This prevents histologic analysis, thereby leading to a risk of understaging of the tumor.

Both types of laser offer good functional and cosmetic outcomes in an outpatient setting, with studies suggesting that combination lasers applied in cases of low-grade tumors produce the best results and lowest rates of recurrence.

Mohs micrographic surgery

Mohs micrographic surgery (MMS) is a form of microscopically controlled chemosurgery that can be performed under local anesthetic. It is most suitable for T1a tumors but has been used up to stage T3. As the surgeon excises the tumor, horizontal sections of all margins are fixed with zinc chloride or in frozen specimens and sent immediately for microscopy. The direction and location of any further excision in the operation is determined by the presence of positive margins. All further excisions are similarly sent for microscopy until all margins are tumor free.

MMS allows for maximum organ preservation, but concerns about recurrence rates persist. Although reporting a 92% cancer-free survival rate, Shindel and colleagues[9] acknowledged MMS offered only a 68% local control rate after a single procedure, with 8 of their 33 patients suffering with local recurrence. They postulated that this may have been due to inadequate depth margins, with surgeons avoiding deep resections, concerned about the absence of reconstructive

Table 1
Oncological outcomes after glans resurfacing

Study	Tumor Stage	No. of Patients	Recurrence (No Study Found Progression)	Cancer-Specific Survival, %
Ayres et al,[16] 2012	T1a	36	Recurrence: 2	NR
Hadway et al,[11] 2006	CIS	10	Recurrence: 0	100
Hakansson et al,[17] 2015	CIS	12	Recurrence: 0	100
Palminteri,[18] 2007	T1-T2	5	Recurrence: 0	NR
Shabbir et al,[10] 2011	CIS	25	Recurrence: 1	NR
Shabbir et al,[10] 2011	T1a	7	Recurrence: 1	NR

Abbreviations: CIS, carcinoma in situe; NR, not reported.

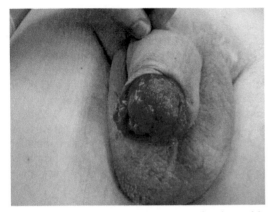

Fig. 1. Superficial squamous cell cancer (SCC) suitable for total glans resurfacing.

urologists at their centers. Concerns regarding recurrence have also been highlighted elsewhere, with Mohs himself acknowledging that distal tumors had much better cure rates, compared with just 57% in cancers with penile shaft involvement. Size, too, has implications, with Mohs citing a 50% cure rate for lesions larger 3 cm.[19,20]

Wide local excision/partial glansectomy

Patients with low-grade, discrete lesions up to T1a can be treated with wide local excisions. In most patients, if the defect is small, primary closure results in only minimal glans deformity. In those with larger lesions, or those close to the urethral meatus, a split skin graft or shaft skin advancement may be required to achieve good cosmetic and functional outcome.

Stage T1b/T2 Tumors Confined to the Glans: Glansectomy

Glansectomy offers the best surgical approach for T2 or high-grade T1 disease (**Table 2**). In this procedure, the glans is separated from the corporal heads and the urethra is not preserved distally

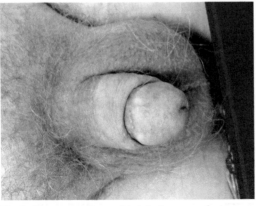

Fig. 2. Three months post total glans resurfacing.

and is instead transected and mobilized such that a urethrostomy is formed at the distal end of the penis accounting for the new penile length. This loss of urethral length makes it an appropriate operation for management of distal urethral tumors.

As in glans resurfacing, the procedure is performed under a general anesthetic with a penile tourniquet in use. A circumferential incision toward Buck fascia is made, 1 cm below the corona. Depending on the location and extension of the penile lesion, a plane of dissection should then be created, before the glans penis is dissected free. Frozen sections from the corpora and distal urethra may be taken if there are concerns about positive margins. For those in whom positive margins are identified, "shaving" of the corporal heads should be performed before any mobilization of the urethra or reconstruction.

If the remaining urethra is too ventrally positioned, spatulation and mobilization of the urethra may be required. Shaft skin is advanced to 2 cm distal to the tip of the penis and the neoglans created using a split-thickness skin graft harvested from the thigh. The graft should include an air dermatome and be between 0.008 and 0.016 in thickness. It should be sutured and quilted with 5 to 0 interrupted vicryl sutures and dressed with a soft paraffin gauze followed by a foam dressing. A catheter should be placed to keep the wound clean and dry and the patient is then placed on 48-hour strict bed rest. The dressing and catheter should be removed on the fifth day before discharge, with a plan for wound review after 1 week.

Proposed by Austoni and colleagues,[24] there is increasing evidence for the glansectomy technique. Patients often have high-risk, invasive cancer, meaning that positive margins are not uncommon. Despite this, Veeratterapillay and colleagues[25] cited only a 13% positive margin rate and a 4% recurrence rate in their cohort of 46 patients. Equally important, all 10 patients in the study by Palminteri and colleagues[18] and all 46 in the study by Veeratterapillay and colleagues[25] reported being satisfied with the appearance of their penis after surgery. Sexual ability is also preserved, although a study by Morelli and colleagues[26] noted that all patients reported sensitivity as being reduced. Complications include graft failure, graft stenosis, and urethral stenosis and are cited at 8% in a cohort of 25 patients[22,23] (**Figs. 5** and **6**).

Stage 2b/Distal T3 Disease: Partial Penectomy/ Distal Corporectomy

For tumors extending into corporal bodies or urethra, partial penectomy offers low recurrence rates

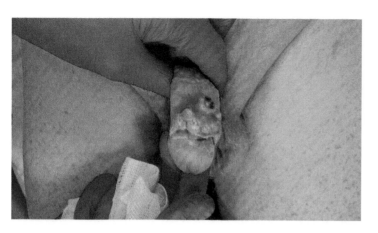

Fig. 3. Superficial inner prepuce tumor with differentiated Penile Intraepithelial Neoplasia (PeIN) extending onto the glans, suitable for partials glans resurfacing.

and, if used in conjunction with reconstructive or lengthening techniques, may offer an acceptable functional and cosmetic outcome (**Table 3**).

Patients should be administered preoperative antibiotics on induction of their general anesthetic, and a penile tourniquet used for control of hemostasis. A circumferential incision 1 to 2 cm proximal to the lesion is made to deglove the penis. This skin should be mobilized to expose the Buck fascia underneath. The corpora and urethra should then be transected proximal to the lesion. This should generate a fish-mouth appearance to the corpora to allow for midline vertical closure. One should be careful to ensure the urethra is 1 cm longer than the corpora to allow for the spatulation required for reconstruction. Successive frozen section biopsies should be sent from the remaining corpora until adequate tumor-free margins are seen before the corpora is closed using 2 to 0 polydioxanone suture. The urethra should then be spatulated dorsally before being sutured circumferentially to the tip of the penis. The penile shaft skin should then be advanced and sutured 2 to 3 cm from the tip of the penis using 4 to 0 interrupted vicryl sutures. To cover the exposed corpora, a neoglans should be created using a split-thickness skin graft harvested from the thigh. The graft should include an air dermatome and be between 0.008 and 0.016 in thickness. It should be sutured and quilted with 5 to 0 interrupted vicryl sutures and dressed with a soft paraffin gauze followed by a foam dressing. A catheter should be placed to keep the wound clean and dry and the patient is then placed on 48-hour strict bed rest. The dressing and catheter should be removed on the fifth day before discharge, with a plan for wound review after 1 week.

As an alternative for those with multiple comorbidities or in whom cosmetic and sexual function is less valued, a skin graft may not be necessary. Instead, shaft skin should be advanced over the corpora and sutured circumferentially around the urethra.

A common concern with partial penectomy is length of the resultant phallus and its implications on potency and urinary function. In some cases, lengthening procedures may be required. This can be achieved by dividing the penile suspensory

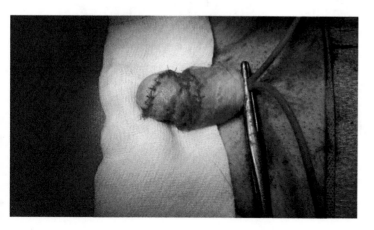

Fig. 4. Intraoperative: after partial glans resurfacing and circumcision.

Table 2
Oncological outcomes after glansectomy

Study	Tumor Stage	No. of Patients	Local Recurrence	Cancer-Specific Survival, %
Gulino et al,[21] 2013	Ta-T3	42	NR	100
Hakansson et al,[17] 2015	T0-T3	15	Recurrence 0	100
Morelli et al,[26] 2009	Ta-T3	15	Recurrence: 0 Metastases (nodal): 1	93.3
O'Kane et al,[22] 2011	T1-T3	25	Recurrence: 1 Metastases (nodal): 2	92
Palminteri,[18] 2007	T1-T2	5	Recurrence: 0	NR
Smith et al,[23] 2007	T1-T2	72	Recurrence: 3	NR

Abbreviation: NR, not reported.

ligament beneath the penile arch and reattaching those to the inferior pubic bone. Alternatively, a scrotoplasty may relieve tethering and traction. Men with large suprapubic fat pads may benefit from liposuction or fat pad excision, whereas in some men a penile prosthesis may be required.

Patients undergoing partial penectomy should be assessed against several outcomes: urinary symptoms, complications, erectile function, patient reported satisfaction, and oncological outcomes. Sansalone and colleagues[30] reported on sexual outcomes, stating that of their 25 patients, 68% were confident in their ability to achieve an erection, 72% were confident of their postoperative potency, and 64% were able to achieve an orgasm. Despite this, all reported less-frequent sex and embarrassment in the size of their penis, a finding reflected by a Dutch study of 90 patients. They compared the patient-reported outcomes of patients undergoing partial penectomy with those who underwent alternative penile-preserving surgery, citing that urinary function, appearance concerns, and orgasm were all much less of a concern

to the latter category.[31] However, oncological outcomes are favorable in partial penectomy, with Rempelakos and colleagues[29] reporting no recurrences in their cohort of 227 patients after 120 months of follow-up.

WHAT IF THE TUMOR/PEIN EXTENDS INTO THE GLANULAR URETHRA?

Extension of penile tumors into the urethra is rare. If the tumor is visible at the urethral meatus, formation of hypospadias, biopsy, and topical treatment may be adequate. For more invasive disease, both partial penectomy and distal corporectomy are viable treatment options, although if remaining penile length is very limited, then a perineal urethrostomy may be required.[32]

At our center, we have investigated the role of substitution urethroplasty for distal urethral tumors concluding that it offers both functional and oncologically effective outcomes. To ensure maximal urethral length, initial excision is done using frozen section. Patients are then offered either a

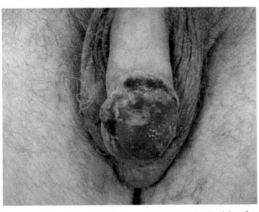

Fig. 5. T2a SCC of glans spongiosus, suitable for glansectomy.

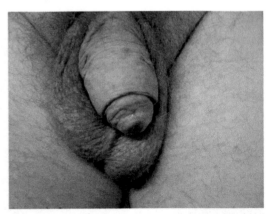

Fig. 6. Postoperative appearance at 3 months after glansectomy.

Table 3
Oncological outcomes after partial penectomy

Study	Tumor Stage	No. of Patients	Recurrence	Mean Follow-up, mo
Korets et al,[27] 2007	Tis-T3; N1-3	32	0	34
Leitje et al,[7] 2008	Tis-T3	214	15	60.6
Ornellas et al,[28] 2008	Ta-T3	522	20	11
Rempelakos et al,[29] 2004	T1-3; N1-3	227	0	>120

synchronous or delayed urethroplasty with buccal graft. In a study of 19 completed surgeries, no patient had suffered local recurrence or urethral strictures at 5 years.[33]

IS THERE A ROLE FOR PENILE-PRESERVING SURGERY IN SALVAGE TREATMENT?

Historically, it was thought that penile-preserving surgery should be avoided in the management of local recurrence after radiotherapy. Recurrence occurs in 30% of patients after radiotherapy and may be difficult to identify due to radiotherapy-related skin change.[34] A study at a supraregional center looked at the management of 17 patients referred to us with chronic ulceration after radiotherapy; 14 of those underwent glansectomy with neoglans formation and at 3 years 13 were disease free.[35] This suggests that penile-preserving surgery may have a role to play in salvage surgery, although further evidence is required.

DOES PENILE-PRESERVING SURGERY AFFECT SURVIVAL?

A persistent concern shrouding penile-preserving surgery is that penile preservation may increase the risk of locoregional recurrence and subsequent associated mortality. Several studies have addressed this hypothesis, with evidence suggesting that between 19% and 29% of patients experience recurrence, a figure much higher than that quoted for patients who undergo partial penectomy.[7–9] Despite that, in a study of 859 patients, no difference in cancer-specific survival was demonstrated between the 2 groups.[24]

SUMMARY

With close follow-up and self-examination, penile-preserving surgery offers an excellent oncological and functional outcome for use in distal penile or urethral malignancy. For more novel techniques, outcome reporting using validated questionnaires is limited; however, it is clear that they offer significantly less psychological and physical morbidity than traditional techniques.

REFERENCES

1. Muneer A, Arya M, Horenblas S. Textbook of penile cancer. Heidelberg: Springer-Verlag London Limited; 2012. p. 126.
2. Hakenberg OW, Watkin N, Comperat E, et al. EAU guidelines on penile cancer: 2014 update. Eur Urol 2015;67(1):142–50.
3. Agrawal A, Pai D, Ananthakrishnan N, et al. The histological extent of the local spread of carcinoma of the penis and its therapeutic implications. BJU Int 2000;85(2):299–301.
4. Minhas S, Kayes O, Hegarty P, et al. What surgical resection margins are required to achieve oncological control in men with primary penile cancer? BJU Int 2005;96(7):1040–3.
5. Hoffman M, Renshaw A, Loughlin KR. Squamous cell carcinoma of the penis and microscopic pathologic margins. How much margin is needed for local cure? Cancer 1999;85(7):1565–8.
6. Hegarty PK, Shabbir M, Hughes B, et al. Penile preserving surgery and surgical strategies to maximize penile form and function in penile cancer: recommendations from the United Kingdom experience. World J Urol 2009;27:179.
7. Leijte JA, Kirrander P, Antonini N, et al. Recurrence patterns of squamous cell carcinoma of the penis: recommendations for follow-up based on a two-centre analysis of 700 patients. Eur Urol 2008; 54(1):161–8.
8. Windahl T, Andersson S-O. Combined laser treatment for penile carcinoma: results after long-term followup. J Urol 2003;169(6):2118–21.
9. Shindel AW, Mann MW, Lev RY, et al. Mohs micrographic surgery for penile cancer: management and long-term followup. J Urol 2007;178(5):1980–5.
10. Shabbir M, Muneer A, Kalsi J, et al. Glans resurfacing for the treatment of carcinoma in situ of the penis: surgical technique and outcomes. Eur Urol 2011;59(1):142–7.
11. Hadway P, Corbishley CM, Watkin NA. Total glans resurfacing for premalignant lesions of the penis: initial outcome data. BJU Int 2006;98(3):532–6.

12. Ekalaksananan T, Pientong C, Thinkhamrop J, et al. Cervical cancer screening in north east Thailand using the visual inspection with acetic acid (VIA) test and its relationship to high-risk human papillomavirus (HR-HPV) status. J Obstet Gynaecol Res 2010 Oct;36(5):1037–43.

13. Kellokoski J, Syrjänen S, Kataja V, et al. Acetowhite staining and its significance in diagnosis of oral mucosal lesions in women with genital HPV infections. J Oral Pathol Med 1990;19(6):278–83.

14. Frega A, French D, Pace S, et al. Prevalence of acetowhite areas in male partners of women affected by HPV and squamous intra-epithelial lesions (SIL) and their prognostic significance. A multicenter study. Anticancer Res 2006;26(4B):3171–4.

15. Depasquale I, Park AJ, Bracka A. The treatment of balanitis xerotica obliterans. BJU Int 2000;86: 459–65.

16. Ayres B, Lam W, Al-Najjar H, et al. Oncological outcomes of glans resurfacing in the treatment of selected superficially invasive penile cancers. J Urol 2012;187(Suppl 4):e306.

17. Håkansson U, Kirrander P, Uvelius B, et al. Organ-sparing reconstructive surgery in penile cancer: initial experiences at two Swedish referral centres. Scand J Urol 2015;49(2):149–54.

18. Palminteri E, Berdondini E, Lazzeri M, et al. Resurfacing and reconstruction of the glans penis. Eur Urol 2007;52(3):893–8.

19. Mohs FE, Snow SN, Larson PO. Mohs micrographic surgery for penile tumours. Urol Clin North Am 1992; 19(2):291–304.

20. Djajadiningrat RS, van Werkhoven E, Meinhardt W, et al. Penile sparing surgery for penile cancer—does it affect survival. J Urol 2014;192(1):120–5.

21. Gulino G, Sasso F, Palermo G, et al. Sexual outcomes after organ potency-sparing surgery and glans reconstruction in patients with penile carcinoma. Indian J Urol 2013;29(2):119–23.

22. O'Kane HF, Pahuja A, Ho KJ, et al. Outcome of glansectomy and skin grafting in the management of penile cancer. Adv Urol 2011;2011:240824.

23. Smith Y, Hadway P, Biedrzycki O, et al. Reconstructive surgery for invasive squamous carcinoma of the glans penis. Eur Urol 2007;52(4):1179–85.

24. Austoni E, Altieri VM, Tenaglia R. Trans-scrotal penile degloving, a new procedure for corporoplasties. Urologia 2012;79(3):200–10.

25. Veeratterapillay R, Sahadevan K, Aluru P, et al. Organ-preserving surgery for penile cancer: description of techniques and surgical outcomes. BJU Int 2012;110(11):1792–5.

26. Morelli G, Pagni R, Mariani C, et al. Glansectomy with split-thickness skin graft for the treatment of penile carcinoma. Int J Impot Res 2009;21(5): 311–4.

27. Korets R, Koppie TM, Snyder ME, et al. Partial penectomy for patients with squamous cell carcinoma of the penis: the Memorial Sloan-Kettering experience. Ann Surg Oncol 2007; 14(12):3614–9.

28. Ornellas AA, Kinchin EW, Nóbrega BL, et al. Surgical treatment of invasive squamous cell carcinoma of the penis: Brazilian National Cancer Institute long-term experience. J Surg Oncol 2008;97(6): 487–95.

29. Rempelakos A, Bastas E, Lymperakis CH, et al. Carcinoma of the penis: experience from 360 cases. J BUON 2004;9(1):51–5.

30. Sansalone S, Silvani M, Leonardi R, et al. Sexual outcomes after partial penectomy for penile cancer: results from a multi-institutional study. Asian J Androl 2015. [Epub ahead of print].

31. Kieffer JM, Djajadiningrat RS, van Muilekom EA, et al. Quality of life for patients treated for penile cancer. J Urol 2014;192(4):1105–10.

32. Smith Y, Hadway P, Ahmed S, et al. Penile-preserving surgery for male distal urethral carcinoma. BJU Int 2007;100(1):82–7.

33. Kulkarni M, Sahu M, Coscione A, et al. Substitution urethroplasty for treatment of distal urethral carcinoma/CIS. Eur Urol Suppl 2015;14(2):E712.

34. Hegarty PK, Eardley I, Heidenreich A, et al. Penile cancer: organ-sparing techniques. BJU Int 2014; 114(6):799–805.

35. Shabbir M, Hughes BE, Swallow T, et al. Management of chronic radiotherapy ulceration after radiotherapy for penile cancer. Eur Urol Suppl 2008;7:112.

Contemporary Role of Radiotherapy in the Management of Primary Penile Tumors and Metastatic Disease

Juanita Crook, MD, FRCPC

KEYWORDS

- Penile cancer • Radiotherapy • Brachytherapy • Surface mold radiotherapy
- Radiotherapy management of regional lymph nodes • Postoperative radiotherapy
- Combined chemoradiotherapy • Penile cancer clinical trials

KEY POINTS

- Squamous cell cancer of the penis is a radiocurable malignancy all too often managed by partial or total penectomy.
- External radiotherapy and brachytherapy have a role to play in the definitive management of the primary tumor, with 5-year penile preservation rates reported at 60% and 85%, respectively.
- Nodal staging remains a cornerstone of management because it is the strongest predictor of survival and inguinal status determines pelvic management.
- Postoperative radiotherapy of the regional nodes for high-risk pathology is indicated.
- Chemoradiotherapy should be considered as neoadjuvant treatment for unresectable nodes or as definitive management.

INTRODUCTION

The vast majority of penile cancers are squamous cell carcinoma (SCC), a radiosensitive and radio curable malignancy. There is consistent evidence across other SCC sites, including head and neck, cervix, vulva, and anal canal, that radiotherapy and the combination of sensitizing chemotherapy and radiotherapy are effective treatment. Furthermore, all these sites share a common pathway in human papillomavirus causation in a significant percentage of cases. Human papillomavirus positivity is associated with a better outcome and higher response rates to chemoradiation, and in penile cancer has been associated with improved 5-year survival.[1,2]

Largely owing to the relative rarity of penile cancer in Western societies, there is a paucity of level 1 evidence to guide treatment. The incidence of approximately 1 per 100,000 in North America and the developed countries of Western Europe is an obstacle to completion of randomized studies to compare surgery with radiotherapy or radiation to chemoradiation.[3]

The traditional surgical approach to penile cancer has been partial or total penectomy. Because of the impact on sexual function, quality of life, and mental health,[4,5] recent advances in surgery toward maximizing penile preservation, such as glansectomy and glans resurfacing, have attempted to address these issues but are not widely

Department of Surgery, Center for the Southern Interior, British Columbia Cancer Agency, 399 Royal Avenue, Kelowna V1Y5L3, British Columbia, Canada
E-mail address: jcrook@bccancer.bc.ca

Urol Clin N Am 43 (2016) 435–448
http://dx.doi.org/10.1016/j.ucl.2016.06.005

adopted.[6,7] There are obvious quality of life advantages to organ preservation that can be provided by nonsurgical alternatives.

In localized disease, various forms of radiotherapy, including external beam, interstitial brachytherapy, and surface mold brachytherapy, offer a high chance of cure with organ preservation, reserving surgery for local recurrence. When there is a significant risk of regional node involvement by virtue of the stage or grade of the primary tumor, management with radiation can be combined with surgical staging of the nodes. The indications for postoperative adjuvant radiation to regional lymphatics following nodal staging are well-established from other anogenital SCC sites and include:

- Multiple node involvement,
- Extracapsular/extranodal extension, and
- Positive surgical margins.

For men presenting with locally and/or regionally advanced disease, chemoradiotherapy may render the disease resectable or can be instituted as a definitive treatment.

RADIOTHERAPY FOR THE PRIMARY TUMOR

Penile preservation should always be considered for the primary tumor. Although not always possible, especially in more locally advanced T3 to T4 disease, quality of life advantages include maintenance of erectile and sexual function and preserved sense of manliness. Delaunay and colleagues[8] published results of a self-reported questionnaire administered to 21 men at an average of 80 months after penile brachytherapy. Seventeen of 18 men potent before brachytherapy reported maintenance of erections and 10 were still in an active sexual relationship. Although the capacity for erection and ejaculation can be maintained after partial penectomy, the lack of a glans and small penile size are cited as reasons for cessation of sexual activity.[9] Emotional and mood disorders, anxiety, depression,[10,11] and even suicide or attempted suicide are reported.[5] Radiation therapy is associated with better global sexual scores than partial penectomy or local excision.[12] An analysis of 128 patients from 6 studies of surgical management of penile carcinoma reported impaired well-being in up to 40%, with psychiatric symptoms in approximately 50%. Additionally, up to 75% of patients report a reduction in sexual function after surgery.[10]

CARCINOMA IN SITU

SCC in situ may be adequately treated with circumcision if confined to the foreskin. Topical therapies such as 5-flouro-uracil cream or imiquoid provide excellent cosmetic results but careful follow-up is mandatory as recurrence is not uncommon. Other penile-sparing options include laser ablation, preferably Nd-YAG lasers, which penetrate up to 6 mm, have shown good tumor control (7% local failure [LF] at 4 years) with satisfactory function and cosmesis; 75% of men resume sexual activity.[13–15] Mohs micrographic surgery or surgical excision with frozen section for intraoperative margin verification may permit local excision, but local recurrence remains a risk after any penile-sparing procedure, reported in up to one-third of patients.[16,17] External beam radiation therapy may be used with a report of 100% local control for in situ disease,[18] but the preferred radiation may be mold plesiotherapy (**Box 1**).

INVASIVE CANCER

Curative radiotherapy of the primary tumor can be delivered either through external beam radiation, interstitial brachytherapy, or surface mold plesiotherapy. For external beam radiotherapy, the 5-year local control and penile preservation rates are about 60%. For low dose rate (LDR) interstitial brachytherapy both local control and penile preservation are about 85% at 5 years and 70% at 10 years.[19,20] Local recurrence is salvageable by surgery and does not affect disease-specific mortality. Each of these modalities is considered in turn.

External Beam Radiotherapy

External beam radiotherapy for early stage localized T1 to T2 SCC of the penis presents challenges with supporting and isolating the organ from adjacent normal structures while positioning it for treatment. Full bolus must be applied to eliminate the skin-sparing characteristics of modern megavoltage beams. With the patient supine, the penis is supported vertically in a split block of tissue-equivalent material with a central chamber to encase the penis (**Fig. 1**). Initially, wax blocks

---

Box 1
Options for squamous cell carcinoma in situ

- Circumcision (if confined to foreskin)
- Topical 5-flouro-uracil/imiquoid
- Nd-YAG laser ablation
- Local excision with margin verification
- External beam radiotherapy
- Surface mold plesiotherapy

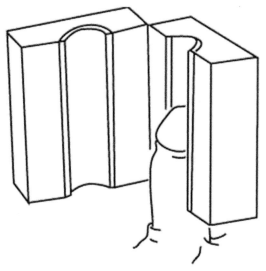

Fig. 1. Bivalved block made of tissue-equivalent material with a central chamber to support the penis during external beam radiotherapy.

penile change over the course of treatment, owing to either swelling or tumor response. With either type of block, it is important to plug the open end with same material to eliminate the air gap distally. Erythema, desquamation, and edema are expected during treatment and take 2 to 4 weeks to heal.

The clinical target volume is the visible/palpable disease with a 1-cm margin. The planned target volume should be a minimum of 2 cm beyond visible/palpable disease to allow for minor setup variation and penumbra. The treated volume includes the full thickness of the penis.

Although dose and fractionation have varied over the decades, currently 66 to 70 Gy over 6.5 to 7 weeks is accepted. Fraction sizes of less than 2 Gy, treatment courses longer than 45 days, and total dose of less than 60 Gy are associated with an increase in local failure.[4,21] The 5-year local control and penile preservation rates range from 41% to 70%[4,18,22–25] with a weighted average of about 61%. Most local failures are salvaged surgically with either partial or total penectomy. Results from selected series are presented in **Table 1**.

External beam radiotherapy is most frequently considered in elderly or debilitated patients or those presenting with locoregionally advanced disease where the primary would be treated in contiguity with the nodal regions, including both

were used for this purpose but being opaque, do not allow verification of penile position for setup before each treatment. Alternatively, if Plexiglas or Lucite chambers are used, the chambers can be sterilized and reused, and setup can be visually checked daily. A range of diameters of the central chamber should be available to accommodate

Table 1
Selected published series for external beam radiotherapy

Author	n	Follow-up (mo)	Dose(Gray)/ # fractions	CSS (%)	DFS	LC (%)	Complications	Penile Preservation (%)
Neave et al,[24] 1993	20	36+	50–55/20–22	58	—	70	10% stenosis	—
McLean et al,[18] 1993	26	116	35/10–60/25	69	15/26	62	27% unspecified	100
Ravi et al,[59] 1994	128	83	50–60	—		65	6% necrosis 24% stenosis	—
Sarin et al,[4] 1997	59	62	50–60	66	—	59	3% necrosis 14% stenosis	55
Gotsadze et akl,[25] 2000	155	40	40–60	88	—	65	1% necrosis 7% stenosis	65
Zouhair et al,[21] 2001	23	70	45–74 @ 1.8–2 Gy	—	—	57	10% stenosis	36
Ozsahin et al,[60] 2006	33	62	52	53 at 10 y	—	44	10% stenosis	52
Azrif et al,[22] 2006	41	54	50–52/16	96	51%	62	8% necrosis 29% stenosis	62
Mistry et al,[23] 2007	18	62	50/20–55/16	85	63%	63	2 necrosis 1 stenosis	66

Abbreviations: CSS, cause-specific survival; DFS, disease-free survival; dose, gray/number of fractions; LC, local control.

groins and the pelvis. This topic is addressed further under Regional Radiotherapy.

Interstitial Low-Dose Rate Brachytherapy

LDR interstitial brachytherapy has been successfully used for decades and can deliver the required dose to the target without excessive treatment of the penile shaft, sparing the contralateral glans in lateralized lesions, and without concerns about daily setup.[26]

LDR interstitial brachytherapy is a 1-hour procedure performed using sterile technique under general anesthesia or penile block. The patient is admitted afterward for 4 to 6 days for treatment delivery. After creation of a sterile field, the visible/palpable lesion is delineated with a sterile pen and appropriate margins chosen. An indwelling Foley catheter is inserted and remains for the duration the brachytherapy treatment. The position and spacing of the interstitial needles is chosen to avoid the urethra, and to have the superficial needles within 3 mm of the treated surface. If they are too shallow, skin ulceration and scarring result. A minimum of a 2-plane implant is required (**Fig. 2**). If necessary, a plesiotherapy plane can be added externally on the side of the

cancer with the air gap filled with appropriate bolus material (**Fig. 3**). A guide template is recommended to ensure parallelism and equal spacing, ideally 12 to 18 mm, with the needles and planes being equidistant. Pairs of templates can be predrilled at a range of needle spacings, but a "universal template" with holes drilled every 3 mm allows more flexibility (**Fig. 4**). Once positioned, the needles must be locked in place individually. Historically, dosimetry was calculated based on measurements of spacing and treated lengths, but the current standard depends on a computed tomography scan for reconstruction of the needles, delineation of the target volume, and dose calculation.

The basic rules of geometry of the Paris system of dosimetry should be appreciated to place the needles optimally.[27] In a classic LDR treatment with iridium wire, the length of the treated volume along the axis of the needles is 0.75 of the active length of the wire sources owing to in-drawing of the isodoses distally between the wires. Similarly, the spacing between the needles determines the lateral margin treated beyond the wires (0.27 × spacing; ie, 4 mm for 15 mm spacing). If a stepping source is used from an automated afterloader, such as in pulse dose rate brachytherapy,

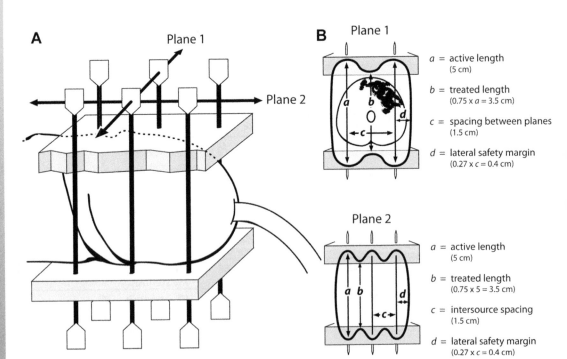

Fig. 2. Two-plane interstitial implant typical of low dose rate brachytherapy and adhering to the Paris rules of dosimetry for geometry and needle spacing. In-drawing of the prescription isodose between the ends of the sources is represented by *b* and the lateral margin around the prescription isodose is shown as *d*. Overview (*A*). Cross sections in Planes 1 and 2 (*B*). (*From* Crook J, Jezioranski J, Cygler JE. Penile brachytherapy: technical aspects and postimplant issues. Brachytherapy 2010;9(2):153; with permission.)

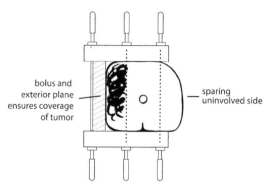

Fig. 3. Schematic of a 3-plane implant showing a plesiotherapy plane of needles exterior to the penis, tissue-equivalent bolus filling the air gap. The depth of needles on the uninvolved side allows skin-sparing on that side. (*From* Crook J, Jezioranski J, Cygler JE. Penile brachytherapy: technical aspects and postimplant issues. Brachytherapy 2010;9(2):156; with permission.)

then dose optimization is possible (**Fig. 5**). The prescribing rules of the Paris system give guidance as to desirable homogeneity, such that dose rate minima between the sources are approximately 115% of the prescription isodose.

Classic continuous LDR brachytherapy aims for a dose rate of 50 to 60 cGy per hour. Pulse dose rate brachytherapy is radiobiologically equivalent if hourly fractions of 0.5 to 0.6 Gy are delivered, 24 hours per day.[28] The total dose recommended is 60 to 65 Gy over 5 days. Minimal analgesia is required, but as many patients are relatively immobile, antithrombotic measures are advised. Needle removal occurs at the bedside after premedication with a narcotic analgesic. Bleeding is usually minimal and the patient can be discharged the same day.

Selected results from the literature are shown in **Table 2**. Five-year local control ranges from 70% to 96% and 10-year from 70% to 80%, with penile preservation at 10 years being 70%. Local failures are salvaged surgically and but may occur late, with 20% occurring up to 8 to 10 years after treatment. Continued surveillance and patient awareness are essential.[19,20,29]

High-Dose Rate Interstitial Brachytherapy

The use of manually afterloaded sources such as iridium 192 wires is no longer available in most departments owing to reasons of staff exposure and the logistics of source disposal after use. In contrast, HDR afterloaders are available in most radiotherapy departments for use in more common malignancies such as breast and prostate, and as an essential component of curative treatment of cervical cancer. Recently, there has been renewed interest in brachytherapy for penile cancer using HDR. The technique is very similar to that described with a few notable exceptions:

1. Needle spacing should be closer than for LDR because HDR is less forgiving of "high-dose sleeves" around sources. Ideal spacing is 9 to 12 mm.
2. Needle spacing does not have to be equidistant because variations in spacing are easily compensated for with the stepping source.
3. A "universal template" with holes every 3 mm is ideal because the spacing around the urethra can be 12 mm and elsewhere reduced to 9 mm
4. Attention to homogeneity is very important. The desired parameters are still being established.

Recent publications indicate that 3 Gy twice daily 6 hours apart is safe and effective for a total

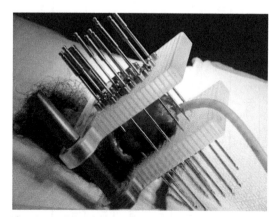

Fig. 4. "Universal" template with holes drilled every 3 mm, so spacing can be selected as suitable at 9, 12, 15, mm and so on; 9 to 12 mm would be suitable for an high dose rate implant whereas 15 mm is the preferred spacing for low dose rate brachytherapy.

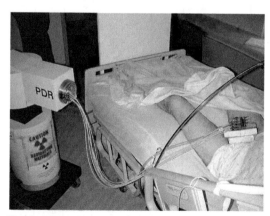

Fig. 5. Patient connected to pulse dose rate machine for pulse dose rate brachytherapy. Fractions are delivered every hour. A Styrofoam plaque distances the treated area from the abdomen.

Table 2
Selected published series for brachytherapy

Author, year	HDR/LDR	n	Follow-up, mo (Range)	Dose, Gray	CSS	DFS	LC	Complications	Penile Preservation
Mazeron et al,[29] 1984	LDR	50	36–96	60–70	79%	63%	78%	3% necrosis 16% stenosis	74%
Delannes et al,[42] 1992	LDR	51	65 (12–144)	50–65	85%	—	86%	23% necrosis 45% stenosis	75%
Rozan et al,[38] 1995	LDR	184	139	59	88% at 5 y; 88 at 10% y	78% at 5 y; 67% at 10 y	85%	21% necrosis 45% stenosis	76%
Soria et al,[5] 1997	LDR	102	111	61–70	72% at 5 y; 66% at 10 y	56% at 5 y; 42% at 10 y	89%	1 necrosis 1 stenosis	68%
Chaudhery et al,[43] 1999	LDR	23	24 (4–117)	50 (40–60)	—	—	70%	0 necrosis 2/23 stenosis	70%
Kiltie et al,[37] 2000	LDR	31	61.5	63.5	85%	85%	81%	8% necrosis 44% stenosis	75%
de Crevoi sier et al,[20] 2009	LDR	144	68 (6–348)	65	92% at 10 y	78% at 10 y	80% at 10 y	26% necrosis 29% stenosis	72% at 10 y
Crook et al,[19] 2009	LDR	67	48 (44–194)	60	84%	71% at 5 y	87% at 5 y; 72% at 10 y	12% necrosis 9% stenosis	88% at 5 y 67% at 10 y
Pimenta et al,[61] 2015	LDR	25	110 (0–228)	60–65 Gy	91%	92% at 5 y crude	1 LF at 4 mo	8% necrosis 43% stenosis	86% at 5 y
Kamsu-Kom et al,[28] 2015	PDR	27	33 (6–64)	60–70	NS	85%	88% at 3 y	9% necrosis 22% stenosis	85%
Petera et al,[31] 2011	HDR	10	20	3 Gy bid = 42–45	100%	NS	100%	0 necrosis 0 stenosis	100%
Sharm et al,[30] 2014	HDR	14	22 (6–40)	3 Gy bid = 51 Gy	83% at 3 y	NS	12/14	0 necrosis 0 stenosis	93%
Rouscoff et al,[34] 2014	HDR	12	27 (5–83)	36/9–39/9 bid	100%	83%	11/12	1/12 necrosis 1/12 stenosis	11/12
Kellas et al,[32] 2015	HDR	55	55 (8–154)	3–3.5 bid = 30–54	NS	NS	73%	0 necrosis 0 stenosis	80%

Abbreviations: CSS, cause-specific survival; DFS, disease-free survival; dose, expressed as range and/or median; HDR, high dose rate; LC, local control; LDR, low dose rate; PDR, pulse dose rate.

dose of 45 to 51 Gy delivered over 7.5 to 8.5 days.[30,31] Penile preservation rates are reported between 80% and 100%. Kellas-Slezka et al[32] report on 55 patients with a median follow-up of 4.5 years. A freehand flexible catheter technique was used to place 2 to 7 catheters in a single (n = 31) or 2-plane (n = 24) implant. Fraction size was 3.0 to 3.5 Gy with a median total dose of 49 Gy after biopsy or 36 Gy after previous total gross excision. Median duration of the implant was 11 days and median follow-up 59 months (range, 8–152). Persistent or recurrent tumors were seen in 11 patients, regional failures in 22%, and distant metastases in 5%. Penile preservation was achieved in 80%. Although this is a large series with mature follow-up, HDR brachytherapy for penile cancer must still be considered to be in evolution; optimal fractionation and homogeneity parameters are yet to be established. Because HDR is less forgiving than LDR, homogeneity parameters are important, with limitation of high-dose volumes within the implant. Greater experience and longer follow-up is required to establish validated guidelines.[33,34]

Surface Mold Plesiotherapy

Originally reported in the LDR era, surface mold plesiotherapy involved an appliance containing iridium wire sources worn for several hours each day for several days to deliver an adequate surface dose with rapid fall-off at a depth.[24] Although initial responses were seen in almost 80% of patients, 45% required subsequent salvage surgery. The dose was low compared with LDR interstitial brachytherapy and a surface mold does not have the benefit of delivering 150% to 200% of the dose to significant intratumoral volumes.

Nonetheless, there is renewed interest in mold plesiotherapy using HDR afterloading with 2 fractions per day, especially for recurrence after laser surgery or topical therapy. Custom molds can be produced with 3-dimensional printing.[35,36] The typical dose is 40 Gy given over 5 days with twice daily fractions of 4 Gy each. With the sources embedded in the mold or applicator at a depth of 5 mm from the skin surface, it is possible to limit the skin dose to approximately 120% of the prescription dose and achieve 100% at an appropriate depth of up to 10 mm, with 90% at a further 5 mm deep (**Fig. 6**). A clear Lucite applicator allows verification of penile position for each fraction. There is minimal swelling or dermatitis at the completion of treatment; the reaction peaks at about 3 weeks and takes 6 to 10 weeks to heal. Because there are no long-term results reported yet, this technique must be considered investigational; however, if efficacy and tolerance are borne out over time, it may well become widely accepted owing to equipment availability and ease of application.

Patient selection

For either interstitial or plesio brachytherapy to tumors involving the glans, circumcision before treatment is essential because it provides full exposure of the lesion; prevents subsequent painful necrosis, phimosis, and fibrosis of the foreskin; and often removes a substantial burden of tumor.

For interstitial brachytherapy, it is recommended that tumors should be confined to the glans and 4 cm or less in maximal diameter.[20,29,37] If there is extension to the coronal sulcus, adequate coverage is obtained with a plane of needles just proximal to the sulcus. Of note, tumor size recommendations are based on limited experience and very small

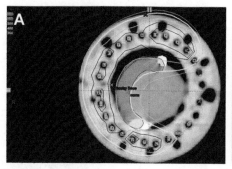 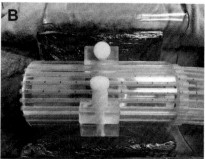

Fig. 6. (*A*) Transverse view of dosimetry through high dose rate (HDR) mold plesiotherapy. Fraction size is 400 cGy, given twice daily with 6 hours between. The 100% isodose is yellow, the surface dose is limited to 120%, and the center receives less than 90% of prescription. The clinical target volume is outlined with wire and is shaded pink. (*B*) HDR plesiotherapy applicator. This is not a custom applicator, but comes in various diameters to suit penile size. The black trough underlying the applicator is a lead shield for the testes. The HDR source is programmed to only treat the required region on the penis; it will only enter the designated transfer tubes and travel the required distance for treatment. The end of the penis fits into the concave surface of a Plexi-glass cork that fills the distal air gap.

numbers of patients in each size category.[29,37] A larger multiinstitutional French experience of 184 patients reported a LF rate of only 20% for tumors greater than 3 cm versus 14% for those 3 cm or smaller (P = .05).[38] Crook and colleagues[39] also reported success with larger tumors in a series of 49 patients with 19 tumors greater than 3 cm, size was not predictive for LF (P = .43). Although both LF and complications such as tissue necrosis are more common with larger tumors, a strict size limit is not appropriate. These selection guidelines should not exclude patients from brachytherapy, especially if the alternative is penectomy, but can provide realistic expectations concerning success of treatment and adverse effects.

Tumor grade does not impact local control with brachytherapy. In the 74 cases reported by Crook and colleagues,[19] one-half were well-differentiated and one-half were moderately or poorly differentiated. Six of 8 local recurrences occurred in well-differentiated cases, whereas only 2 were in moderately or poorly differentiated tumors. However, high-grade lesions are associated with a higher rate of metastatic and regional failure; the status of the regional nodes must be addressed with both imaging and either sentinel lymph node biopsy or groin dissection (**Box 2**).

Similar to considerations for tumor size, the risk of LF increases with tumor stage, being up to 23% to 29% for T3 tumors.[29,38,40,41]

Plesio brachytherapy should be limited to superficial tumors (Tis, T1a or b) and should not be used for those invading the corpus spongiosum or thicker than 5 mm. The same requirement for circumcision holds.

> **Box 2**
> **Indications for surgical node staging**
>
> - Moderate or poor differentiation
> - Lymphovascular invasion
> - Stage T2 or greater

Aftercare

Both interstitial and plesio brachytherapy will cause moist desquamation (**Fig. 7**), which peaks at about 3 weeks and heals in 6 to 10 weeks for plesiotherapy, but may take 2 to 3 months after interstitial brachytherapy. Tumor resolution results in tissue ulceration, the depth of which corresponds with the depth of invasion of the tumor, often leaving a punched-out crater. Biopsy should be reserved for cases suspicious for local recurrence owing to induration or an exophytic component. Healing is much slower in diabetics. Local hygiene is important with frequent

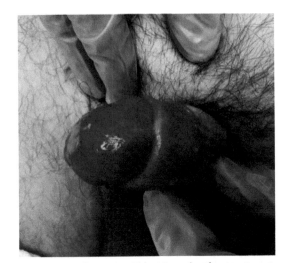

Fig. 7. Moist desquamation at 6 weeks after treatment.

daily soaks in warm water with baking soda or salt. Bacitracin zinc/polymyxin B sulfate (Polysporin) or silver sulfadiazine (Flamazine) can be applied after each soak. Oral antibiotics are not usually necessary. Meatal adhesions, causing a restricted or deviated urinary stream, should be separated using either the tip of a catheter or a meatal dilator. Patients can be given their own dilator after their first visit with instructions on how and when to use it.

Late Toxicity

The most common late sequellae are meatal stenosis and soft tissue ulceration. Skin changes are generally acceptable with minor hypo or hyper pigmentation or telangiectasia (**Fig. 8**).

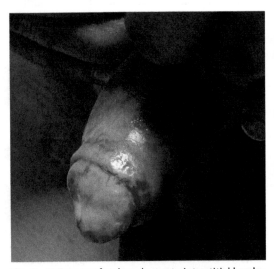

Fig. 8. At 7 years after low dose rate interstitial brachytherapy and bilateral inguinal lymph node dissection for T2 squamous cell carcinoma. Mild hypopigmentation and telangiectasia visible. The patient remained potent.

Meatal stenosis is reported in 9% to 45%[19,20,29,37,38,42] and increases with doses over 60 Gy (LDR interstitial) and with proximity of the needles to the meatus.[38] Stenoses occur relatively late, but usually before 3 years. Many are low grade and can be managed with self-dilatation; meatoplasty or reconstructive surgery are rarely necessary.[29]

Soft tissue ulceration is reported in 0% to 26% of patients after LDR interstitial brachytherapy,[19,20,29,38,42,43] with the higher rates being seen with larger volume implants (≥3 planes), larger and more deeply invasive tumors,[29] and doses >60 Gy.[38] Most will heal over 3 to 6 months with attention to local hygiene, and topical antibiotics. Hydrogen peroxide, topical vitamin E, and topical steroids can also be beneficial. Deeper lesions will respond to a course of hyperbaric oxygen, requiring 30 to 40 "dives" at 2 to 2.5 atm breathing 100% oxygen for 90 minutes[44] (**Fig. 9**).

Regional Radiotherapy

Prophylactic radiation of the inguinal regions for patients at high risk of node involvement by virtue of moderate or poor differentiation, lymphovascular invasion, or stage T2 or greater[45,46] is not generally recommended. Surgical staging is the preferred approach because lymph node status is the most important prognostic factor for survival, and groin node status determines subsequent pelvic management.[47] Therapeutic node dissection performed for nodal failure is much less efficacious than prophylactic/diagnostic dissection.

After inguinal node dissection, the same guidelines for postoperative radiotherapy should be followed as for SCC of the vulva: multiple node involvement or extracapsular/extranodal extension. If the pelvic nodes are known to be clear pathologically, the radiotherapy can be limited to the inguinal region but for a high-risk groin with unknown pelvic node status, the pelvis should be included to a dose of 45 Gy in 25 fractions over 5 weeks. The dose to the groin depends on the extent of the dissection and the presence of positive margins or extracapsular disease in which case a boost to 54 to 63 Gy should be considered (**Box 3**).

COMBINED CHEMORADIOTHERAPY

The evidence for combined chemoradiotherapy in other SCC sites is well-established through multiple mature randomized trials showing improved locoregional control and organ preservation in advanced head and neck SCC,[48] locally advanced anal canal SCC,[49] and improved disease free and overall survival with combined weekly platinum and radiotherapy for cervical SCC.[50]

Vulvar cancer is the SCC site most commonly compared with penile cancer because of the similarities in histopathology, lymph node drainage, population age, and human papillomavirus etiology. In 1986, Homesley and colleagues[51] reported a survival advantage for postoperative groin-plus-pelvic radiotherapy after radical vulvectomy with inguinal node metastases. One hundred fourteen women were randomized to either pelvic lymph node dissection (n = 55) or groin-plus-pelvic radiotherapy (n = 59; 45–50 Gy in 4.5–6 weeks). Pelvic-plus-groin radiotherapy showed a 14% increase in 2-year survival, from 54% to 68% (P = .02) compared with pelvic node dissection. Groin failures were reduced

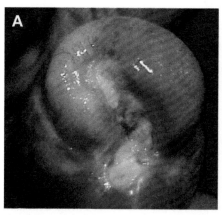
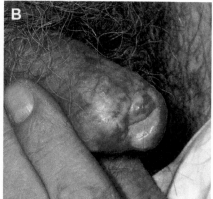

Fig. 9. (*A*) Tissue necrosis after low dose rate brachytherapy for a T3 squamous cell carcinoma (invading the ventral urethra) in a 47-year-old man. (*B*) Healed after hyperbaric oxygen. Results at 5 years. The patient remained potent.

from 13 of 55 to 3 of 59. If 2 or more lymph nodes were involved, the survival improvement increased from 37% to 63%.

A subsequent trial used preoperative combined chemoradiotherapy for advanced vulvar cancer.[52] Treatment consisted of 4760 cGy in split course with cisplatinum 50 mg/m^2 and 5FU. In 38 of 40 patients with N2-3 SCC of the vulva, the nodes became resectable and a complete histologic response was seen in 15 patients.

The next trial for advanced vulvar cancer used a continuous course of radiotherapy to 57.6 Gy plus

weekly platinum at a dose of 40 mg/m^2, as per the cervical cancer standard.[53] In 58 women with unresectable locally advanced T3 to T4 SCC, complete response was documented by biopsy in 64%. Forty-seven percent of the women were older than 60 years and 24% were older than 70. These trials all used very simple radiotherapy beam arrangements; however, subsequently intensity modulated radiation therapy with combined chemotherapy has been used for stage II to IVa vulvar cancer, with excellent tolerance and no grade 3 or higher toxicity in 18 patients.[54]

From this series of sequential clinical trials on vulvar cancer, current management of locoregionally advanced disease has been defined as a continuous course of radiotherapy in 1.8 Gy daily fractions to a dose of 57.6 Gy, combined with weekly cisplatinum at 40 mg/m^2. Intensity modulated radiation therapy is recommended to decrease toxicity. The American College of Radiology Appropriateness Criteria for the management of locoregionally advanced SCC of the

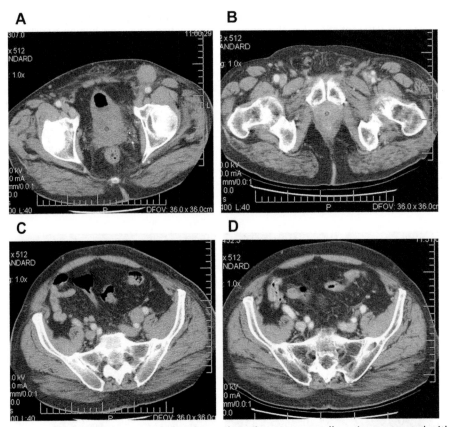

Fig. 10. A 76-year-old man with locoregionally advanced penile squamous cell carcinoma treated with external beam radiotherapy and concurrent weekly cisplatinum. Computed tomography scans showing baseline (*A, B*) left inguinal adenopathy and (*C, D*) left iliac adenopathy and response respectively at 3 months following chemoradiotherapy.

vulva specifically recommend either neoadjuvant chemoradiotherapy or definitive chemoradiation.[55] Only in countries where radiation therapy is not available would neoadjuvant chemotherapy alone be considered an option.

The weight of evidence from other SCC sites would suggest a similar approach for penile cancer. Currently, the International Rare Cancers Initiative, Cancer Research UK, the Institute of Cancer Research, and the National Cancer Institute are collaborating in InPACT (International Penile Advanced Cancer Trial), hoping to define the role of neoadjuvant therapy. Using a Bayesian design, 400 patients from Europe and the United States will be accrued over a 5-year period. For node-positive penile cancer, surgery will be compared with neoadjuvant chemotherapy and neoadjuvant chemoradiotherapy. For those men with a high risk of pelvic node involvement, prophylactic pelvic lymph node dissection followed when indicated by chemoradiation will be compared with chemoradiation alone, without surgery to the pelvis.[56]

Until such time as InPACT provides the required evidence, following the lead from other SCC sites including vulvar SCC and cervical cancer, the combination radiotherapy plus weekly cisplatinum at a dose of 40 mg/m^2 is recommended for locoregionally advanced penile cancer not considered operable. This approach is well-tolerated and effective even in elderly patients, provided they have adequate renal function.[50,57] If response to treatment renders the disease resectable, this can be planned after a dose of 45 Gy, the alternative being to continue to a definitive dose for the bulk of disease, bearing in mind that lower radiation doses will be effective when combined with weekly cisplatin. **Figs. 10** and **11** illustrate the application of this approach.

Palliative Treatment

Standard short course radiotherapy of a single, 5, or 10 fractions may palliate metastatic disease but is not highly effective for bulky groin adenopathy. Although these patients may be elderly and frail, consideration should be given to combined platinum and radiotherapy provided kidney function is adequate with a glomerular filtration rate in excess of 50 mL/min.

SUMMARY

Although penile preservation is recognized as an important goal, penile cancer is relatively uncommon and largely managed in the community where urologic surgeons may not be experienced

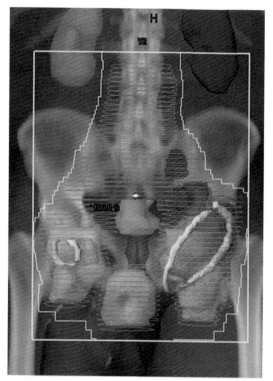

Fig. 11. Treatment fields with adenopathy contoured on computed tomography and outlined with wire in the inguinal regions. The entire volume received 4500 cGy in 25 fractions over 5 weeks, followed by a boost to the right groin to 5500 cGy and to the left groin to 6500 cGy. Cisplatinum was given at 40 mg/m^2 weekly.

in surgical alternatives to penectomy. Radiotherapy is widely accessible and can provide an effective penile-sparing alternative. A recent metaanalysis by Hasan and colleagues[58] looked at the outcome of surgery compared with brachytherapy for 2178 men, 1505 treated by penectomy and 673 by brachytherapy. Organ preservation for brachytherapy was 74%. For stage I or II disease, the 5-year overall survival was 80% for surgery (n = 659) and 79% for brachytherapy (n = 209) and local control was 86% versus 84%. Despite these excellent results, urologists are not always aware that the radiotherapy option should be considered.

Radiotherapy has a clear role to play in the curative management of SCC of the penis, both in management of the primary tumor and in control of the high-risk groin or pelvis after surgical nodal staging. Acceptance of the latter is growing and the success of InPACT will provide much needed level 1 evidence.

REFERENCES

1. Lont AP, Kroon BK, Horenblas S, et al. Presence of high-risk human papillomavirus DNA in penile carcinoma predicts favorable outcome in survival. Int J Cancer 2006;119(5):1078–81.

2. Djajadiningrat RS, Jordanova ES, Kroon BK, et al. Human papillomavirus prevalence in invasive penile cancer and association with clinical outcome. J Urol 2015;193(2):526–31.

3. Hernandez BY, Barnholtz-Sloan J, German RR, et al. Burden of invasive squamous cell carcinoma of the penis in the United States, 1998-2003. Cancer 2008;113(10 Suppl):2883–91.

4. Sarin R, Norman AR, Steel GG, et al. Treatment results and prognostic factors in 101 men treated for squamous carcinoma of the penis. Int J Radiat Oncol Biol Phys 1997;38(4):713–22.

5. Soria JC, Fizazi K, Piron D, et al. Squamous cell carcinoma of the penis: multivariate analysis of prognostic factors and natural history in monocentric study with a conservative policy. Ann Oncol 1997; 8(11):1089–98.

6. Philippou P, Shabbir M, Malone P, et al. Conservative surgery for squamous cell carcinoma of the penis: resection margins and long-term oncological control. J Urol 2012;188(3):803–8.

7. Shabbir M, Muneer A, Kalsi J, et al. Glans resurfacing for the treatment of carcinoma in situ of the penis: surgical technique and outcomes. Eur Urol 2011;59(1):142–7.

8. Delaunay B, Soh PN, Delannes M, et al. Brachytherapy for penile cancer: Efficacy and impact on sexual function. Brachytherapy 2014; 13(4):380–7.

9. Romero FR, Romero KR, Mattos MA, et al. Sexual function after partial penectomy for penile cancer. Urology 2005;66(6):1292–5.

10. Maddineni SB, Lau MM, Sangar VK. Identifying the needs of penile cancer sufferers: a systematic review of the quality of life, psychosexual and psychosocial literature in penile cancer. BMC Urol 2009;9:8.

11. Ficarra V, D'Amico A, Cavalleri S, et al. Surgical treatment of penile carcinoma: our experience from 1976 to 1997. Urol Int 1999;62(4):234–7.

12. Opjordsmoen S, Waehre H, Aass N, et al. Sexuality in patients treated for penile cancer: patients' experience and doctors' judgement. Br J Urol 1994;73(5): 554–60.

13. Windahl T, Andersson SO. Combined laser treatment for penile carcinoma: results after long-term followup. J Urol 2003;169(6):2118–21.

14. Windahl T, Skeppner E, Andersson SO, et al. Sexual function and satisfaction in men after laser treatment for penile carcinoma. J Urol 2004; 172(2):648–51.

15. Frimberger D, Hungerhuber E, Zaak D, et al. Penile carcinoma. Is Nd:YAG laser therapy radical enough? J Urol 2002;168(6):2418–21 [discussion: 2421].

16. Mohs FE, Snow SN, Larson PO. Mohs micrographic surgery for penile tumors. Urol Clin North Am 1992; 19(2):291–304.

17. Shindel AW, Mann MW, Lev RY, et al. Mohs micrographic surgery for penile cancer: management and long-term followup. J Urol 2007;178(5): 1980–5.

18. McLean M, Akl AM, Warde P, et al. The results of primary radiation therapy in the management of squamous cell carcinoma of the penis. Int J Radiat Oncol Biol Phys 1993;25(4):623–8.

19. Crook J, Ma C, Grimard L. Radiation therapy in the management of the primary penile tumor: an update. World J Urol 2009;27(2):189.

20. de Crevoisier R, Slimane K, Sanfilippo N, et al. Long-term results of brachytherapy for carcinoma of the penis confined to the glans (N- or NX). Int J Radiat Oncol Biol Phys 2009;74(4): 1150–6.

21. Zouhair A, Coucke PA, Jeanneret W, et al. Radiation therapy alone or combined surgery and radiation therapy in squamous-cell carcinoma of the penis? Eur J Cancer 2001;37(2): 198–203.

22. Azrif M, Logue JP, Swindell R, et al. External-beam radiotherapy in T1-2 N0 penile carcinoma. Clin Oncol (R Coll Radiol) 2006;18(4):320–5.

23. Mistry T, Jones RW, Dannatt E, et al. A 10-year retrospective audit of penile cancer management in the UK. BJU Int 2007;100(6):1277–81.

24. Neave F, Neal AJ, Hoskin PJ, et al. Carcinoma of the penis: a retrospective review of treatment with iridium mould and external beam irradiation. Clin Oncol (R Coll Radiol) 1993;5(4):207–10.

25. Gotsadze D, Matveev B, Zak B, et al. Is conservative organ-sparing treatment of penile carcinoma justified? Eur Urol 2000;38(3):306–12.

26. Crook J, Jezioranski J, Cygler JE. Penile brachytherapy: technical aspects and postimplant issues. Brachytherapy 2010;9(2):151–8.

27. Pierquin B, Chassagne D, Wilson F. Modern brachytherapy. New York: Masoom Pub; 1987.

28. Kamsu-Kom L, Bidault F, Mazeron R, et al. Clinical experience with pulse dose rate brachytherapy for conservative treatment of penile carcinoma and comparison with historical data of low dose rate brachytherapy. Clin Oncol (R Coll Radiol) 2015; 27(7):387–93.

29. Mazeron JJ, Langlois D, Lobo PA, et al. Interstitial radiation therapy for carcinoma of the penis using iridium 192 wires: the Henri Mondor experience (1970-1979). Int J Radiat Oncol Biol Phys 1984; 10(10):1891–5.

30. Sharma DN, Joshi NP, Gandhi AK, et al. High-dose-rate interstitial brachytherapy for T1-T2-stage penile carcinoma: short-term results. Brachytherapy 2014; 13(5):481–7.

31. Petera J, Sirak I, Kasaova L, et al. High-dose rate brachytherapy in the treatment of penile carcinoma–first experience. Brachytherapy 2011;10(2): 136–40.

32. Kellas-Sleczka S, Bialis B, Fijalkowski M, et al. Interstitial HDR brachytherapy for penile cancer: a 13 year follow up of 55 patients. Brachytherapy 2015; 14(3 S(1)):S33.

33. Crook JM, Keyes M, Dubai R, et al. Lessons learned in converting from a low dose rate to high dose rate penile brachytherapy program. Brachytherapy 2016;16(3 Suppl 1):S86.

34. Rouscoff Y, Falk AT, Durand M, et al. High-dose rate brachytherapy in localized penile cancer: short-term clinical outcome analysis. Radiat Oncol 2014;9:142.

35. Matys R, Kubicka-Mendak I, Lyczek J, et al. Penile cancer brachytherapy HDR mould technique used at the Holycross Cancer Center. J Contemp Brachytherapy 2011;3(4):224–9.

36. Helou J, Morton G, Easton H, et al. Customized penile plesiobrachytherapy using latest stereolithography techniques. Brachytherapy 2015; 14(3 suppl 1):599.

37. Kiltie AE, Elwell C, Close HJ, et al. Iridium-192 implantation for node-negative carcinoma of the penis: the Cookridge Hospital experience. Clin Oncol (R Coll Radiol) 2000;12(1):25–31.

38. Rozan R, Albuisson E, Giraud B, et al. Interstitial brachytherapy for penile carcinoma: a multicentric survey (259 patients). Radiother Oncol 1995;36(2): 83–93.

39. Crook JM, Jezioranski J, Grimard L, et al. Penile Brachytherapy: Results for 49 patients. Int J Radiat Oncol Biol Phys 2005;62(2):460–7.

40. Sobin LH, Gospodarowicz MK, Wittekind C, et al, International Union against Cancer. TNM classification of malignant tumours. 7th 2009 ed. Chichester (United Kingdom): Wiley-Blackwell; 2010.

41. Hermanek P, Sobin LH. TNM classification of malignant tumours, 4th edition. Penis (ICD-0 187). 4th edition. Berlin: Springer-Verlag; 1987.

42. Delannes M, Malavaud B, Douchez J, et al. Iridium-192 interstitial therapy for squamous cell carcinoma of the penis. Int J Radiat Oncol Biol Phys 1992;24(3): 479–83.

43. Chaudhary AJ, Ghosh S, Bhalavat RL, et al. Interstitial brachytherapy in carcinoma of the penis. Strahlenther Onkol 1999;175(1):17–20.

44. Gomez-Iturriaga A, Crook J, Evans W, et al. The efficacy of hyperbaric oxygen therapy in the treatment of medically refractory soft tissue necrosis after penile brachytherapy. Brachytherapy 2011;10(6): 491–7.

45. Solsona E, Algaba F, Horenblas S, et al, European Association of Urology. EAU guidelines on penile cancer. Eur Urol 2004;46(1):1–8.

46. Souillac I, Avances C, Camparo P, et al. Penile cancer in 2010: update from the Oncology Committee of the French Association of Urology: external genital organs group (CCAFU-OGE). Prog Urol 2011; 21(13):909–16.

47. Lont AP, Kroon BK, Gallee MP, et al. Pelvic lymph node dissection for penile carcinoma: extent of inguinal lymph node involvement as an indicator for pelvic lymph node involvement and survival. J Urol 2007;177(3):947–52 [discussion: 952].

48. Forastiere AA, Zhang Q, Weber RS, et al. Long-term results of RTOG 91-11: a comparison of three nonsurgical treatment strategies to preserve the larynx in patients with locally advanced larynx cancer. J Clin Oncol 2013;31(7):845–52.

49. Bartelink H, Roelofsen F, Eschwege F, et al. Concomitant radiotherapy and chemotherapy is superior to radiotherapy alone in the treatment of locally advanced anal cancer: results of a phase III randomized trial of the European Organization for Research and Treatment of Cancer Radiotherapy and Gastrointestinal Cooperative Groups. J Clin Oncol 1997;15(5):2040–9.

50. Stehman FB, Ali S, Keys HM, et al. Radiation therapy with or without weekly cisplatin for bulky stage 1B cervical carcinoma: follow-up of a Gynecologic Oncology Group trial. Am J Obstet Gynecol 2007; 197(5):503.e1-e6.

51. Homesley HD, Bundy BN, Sedlis A, et al. Radiation therapy versus pelvic node resection for carcinoma of the vulva with positive groin nodes. Obstet Gynecol 1986;68(6):733–40.

52. Montana GS, Thomas GM, Moore DH, et al. Preoperative chemo-radiation for carcinoma of the vulva with N2/N3 nodes: a gynecologic oncology group study. Int J Radiat Oncol Biol Phys 2000; 48(4):1007–13.

53. Moore DH, Thomas GM, Montana GS, et al. Preoperative chemoradiation for advanced vulvar cancer: a phase II study of the Gynecologic Oncology Group. Int J Radiat Oncol Biol Phys 1998;42(1):79–85.

54. Beriwal S, Coon D, Heron DE, et al. Preoperative intensity-modulated radiotherapy and chemotherapy for locally advanced vulvar carcinoma. Gynecol Oncol 2008;109(2):291–5.

55. Expert Panel on Radiation Oncology-Gynecology, Kidd E, Moore D, et al. ACR Appropriateness Criteria(R) management of locoregionally advanced squamous cell carcinoma of the vulva. Am J Clin Oncol 2013;36(4):415–22.

56. Barber J. The development of a clinical trial protocol to test the timing and effectiveness of adjuvant and neoadjuvant therapy in locally advanced penile cancer. Curr Probl Cancer 2015;39(3):173–85.

57. Moore DH, Ali S, Koh WJ, et al. A phase II trial of radiation therapy and weekly cisplatin chemotherapy for the treatment of locally-advanced squamous cell carcinoma of the vulva: a gynecologic oncology group study. Gynecol Oncol 2012;124(3):529–33.

58. Hasan S, Francis A, Hagenauer A, et al. The role of brachytherapy in organ preservation for penile cancer: A meta-analysis and review of the literature. Brachytherapy 2015;14(4):517–24.

59. Ravi R, Chaturvedi HK, Sastry DV. Role of radiation therapy in the treatment of carcinoma of the penis. Br J Urol 1994;74(5):646–51.

60. Ozsahin M, Jichlinski P, Weber DC, et al. Treatment of penile carcinoma: to cut or not to cut? Int J Radiat Oncol Biol Phys 2006;66(3):674–9.

61. Pimenta A, Gutierrez C, Mosquera D, et al. Penile brachytherapy-Retrospective review of a single institution. Brachytherapy 2015;14(4):525–30.

Minimal Invasive Management of Lymph Nodes

S. Horenblas, MD, PhD, FEBU[a],*, S. Minhas, MD, FRCS (Urol)[b]

KEYWORDS

- Lymph nodes • Sentinel node • Metastasis • Staging

KEY POINTS

- Early detection of lymph mode involvement is mandatory, as lymph node involvement in men with penile carcinoma is the most important factor determining survival.
- Approximately 10% to 20% of clinically node-negative patients will harbor occult metastases, which are not detectable on conventional cross-sectional imaging.
- Early resection of the inguinal lymph nodes is associated with a therapeutic benefit, and it is imperative that patients with metastatic disease in the inguinal lymph nodes undergo early inguinal lymphadenectomy.
- Dynamic sentinel biopsy has evolved as a reliable minimally invasive staging technique with an associated sensitivity of 85% to 95% together with a low morbidity for the detection of occult metastasis and should be undertaken as the diagnostic staging modality of choice in men with high-risk clinically node-negative disease.

INTRODUCTION

The presence of nodal involvement is the single most important prognostic factor determining survival of penile carcinoma.[1–8] The currently available noninvasive staging modalities have a low sensitivity in detecting small metastatic load, the optimal management of clinically node-negative patients has been the subject of much debate.[9] Approximately 10% to 20% of clinically node-negative patients have occult metastasis. Some clinicians manage these patients with close surveillance. Other diagnostic approaches utilized are dynamic sentinel node biopsy, modified lymphadenectomy, and radical inguinal lymphadenectomy in those patients considered to be at high risk for occult metastases, the so-called risk-adapted approach.[10] Although close surveillance may lead to unintentional delay because of growth and spread of occult metastases in 10% to 20% of clinically node-negative patients, elective inguinal lymphadenectomy and risk-adapted inguinal lymphadenectomy are considered unnecessary in 80% to 90% of such cases because of the absence of metastases.[11,12] Furthermore, lymphadenectomy is associated with significant surgical morbidity and long-term sequelae, including chronic lymphodema. Up to 35% to 70% of patients have short- or long-term complications.[13–16] This article focuses on minimally invasive staging of lymph nodes in men with penile cancer.

ASSESSMENT OF INGUINAL LYMPH NODES

The key issue in lymph node staging is the unreliability of the currently available modalities, which detect occult nodal involvement. However, given that early resection of the inguinal lymph nodes

The authors have nothing to disclose.
a Department of Urology, Netherlands Cancer Institute, Plesmanlaan 121, Amsterdam 1066CX, The Netherlands;
b University College Hospital, London, UK
* Corresponding author.
E-mail address: s.horenblas@nki.nl

Urol Clin N Am 43 (2016) 449–456
http://dx.doi.org/10.1016/j.ucl.2016.06.006

is associated with a therapeutic benefit, it is imperative that those patients with metastatic disease in the inguinal lymph nodes undergo an inguinal lymphadenectomy at the earliest possible time.[17–19] Unfortunately the morbidity associated with an elective inguinal lymphadenectomy includes the operation for every clinically node-negative penile cancer patient. Adopting this approach would overtreat the majority (greater than 80%) of patients with its associated significant morbidity.

CLINICAL EXAMINATION OF THE NODES

Most patients diagnosed with penile cancer in Western countries present without any palpable abnormalities in the groins, and only 10% to 20% of patients present with palpable nodes.[20] Inguinal lymph nodes that become palpable during follow-up are caused by metastasis in nearly 100% of cases.[21] Physical examination of the inguinal region is of limited value, especially in the detection of small metastases. More recently, the diagnostic accuracy of clinical examination has been shown to have a sensitivity of 73%.[22] Approximately 10% to 20% of clinically node-negative patients will harbor occult metastases.[5,23,24] These occult metastases are, by definition, not detectable by physical examination. In clinically node-positive patients, up to 75% of patients will actually have metastatic inguinal nodal involvement,[23] with the remainder having enlarged inguinal nodes secondary to infection associated with the primary tumor.

The currently available noninvasive staging techniques, which can be used to stage the groin besides physical examination, include ultrasonography combined with fine-needle aspiration cytology (FNAC) of suspicious nodes, computed tomography (CT) scan, MRI, and positron emission tomography (PET)/CT-scanning.

ULTRASOUND WITH FINE-NEEDLE ASPIRATION CYTOLOGY

Ultrasound is a simple, noninvasive, and inexpensive imaging modality that can be easily be combined with FNAC for the detection and diagnosis of abnormal-looking lymph nodes. In a series of 43 patients with 83 clinically node-negative groins, ultrasound-guided FNAC had a sensitivity and specificity of 39% and 100%, respectively.[25] Ultrasound-guided FNAC can be used preoperatively to screen the clinically node-negative groin and to further analyze the groins of patients with palpable inguinal lymph nodes. Especially in clinically node-positive patients, FNAC performs well, with a sensitivity and specificity of 93% and 91%, respectively.[26] False-negative rates for FNAC have been reported in up to 15% of cases. If the clinician remains suspicious, repeat FNAC is indicated, and if still inconclusive, excisional biopsy can be performed.

COMPUTED TOMOGRAPHY IMAGING

The role of CT in staging the inguinal lymph nodes is poorly understood due to a paucity of studies. One report published in 1991 described a small series of 14 patients who underwent preoperative CT scanning.[27] Sensitivity and specificity of 36% and 100% were found, respectively. None of the occult metastases in clinically node-negative groins were identified. However, these results are a reflection of the CT technology available at the time of the study. Currently with the use of multislice CT-scanners and increased spatial resolution, results are probably better. Nevertheless, the problem of missing a small metastasis remains. The diagnostic accuracy in the detection of the pelvic lymph nodes is poor, in accordance with the experience recently reported by other centers.[28] Therefore, CT imaging is not recommended as the initial staging tool for clinically node-negative patients, although it may be helpful in those who are difficult to examine (eg, obese patients). In contrast, CT scanning can be useful in clinically node-positive patients to determine size of metastases, the extent of disease, central nodal necrosis, and/or an irregular nodal border. All these factors are strongly associated with an unfavorable prognosis.[29]

MAGNETIC RESONANCE IMAGING

MRI with lymphotrophic nanoparticles (LN-MRI, ultrasmall particles of iron oxide, USPIOs, ferrumoxtran-10) has shown promising results in identifying occult metastases in a study of 7 patients with penile cancer.[30] MRI was performed before and also 24 hours after intravenous ferrumoxtran-10 administration. In this small series, LN-MRI has shown a sensitivity of 100% and a specificity of 97%. This imaging technique has also revealed high diagnostic accuracies in staging lymph nodes in prostate cancer and bladder cancer.[31] However, ferrumoxtran-10 is not approved by the US Food and Drug Administration (FDA); hence it is not currently available. In addition, conventional MRI is also limited by its spatial resolution. Thus, its use is also limited for staging microscopic invasion in the groin.

POSITRON EMISSION TOMOGRAPHY/ COMPUTED TOMOGRAPHY SCAN

PET scanning detects subnanomolar concentrations of radioactive tracer in vivo. Following malignant transformation, a range of tumors can be characterized by elevated glucose metabolism and subsequent increased uptake of the intravenously injected radiolabeled glucose analogue [^{18}F]-fluorodeoxyglucose (FDG). PET scanning combined with low-dose CT imaging (PET/CT) in a single scanner fuses the acquired data into 1 image containing both functional and anatomic information. The accuracy of the combined images is reported to be higher than separate PET and CT images.[32–34]

In 2005, Scher and colleagues[35] published the first results of PET/CT scanning in penile cancer with promising results, a sensitivity of 80% and specificity of 100%. However, in a study of 42 clinically node-negative groins, PET/CT missed 1 out of 5 occult metastases. In addition, 3 false-positive results were found among the 37 remaining groins, leading to a specificity of 92%.[36] The false-positive findings were associated with inflammation in the lymph nodes.

Sadeghi and colleagues[37] systematically reviewed FDG-PET/CT scanning for penile cancer and found a pooled overall sensitivity and specificity of 81% and 92%, respectively. In clinically positive groins these numbers increased to 96% sensitivity and 57% specificity. The limitations of MRI with respect to spatial resolution are also true for PET/CT.

In summary, each of the previously mentioned techniques is not reliable enough in assessing the clinically node-negative patient because of a limited spatial resolution of at least 2 mm. Consequently, false-negative findings (ie, missing small metastases) are inevitable with the currently available noninvasive staging techniques. Furthermore, it is important to emphasize that reported diagnostic accuracies are partly a reflection of patient selection, with lower sensitivities reported when only clinically node-negative patients are studied. Furthermore, CT and MRI have other additional disadvantages, including nonspecific morphologic characteristics (ie, size and shape of the node). Apart from ultrasound when combined with FNAC, lymph nodes can be falsely labeled as a metastasis as opposed to being abnormal secondary to infection, and none of these imaging modalities provide histopathological evidence apart from ultrasound-guided FNAC.

ASSESSMENT OF THE PELVIC LYMPH NODES

Metastases to the pelvic lymph nodes are found only in conjunction with the presence of inguinal metastases. Skip metastases to the pelvic nodes without inguinal involvement have hardly been documented, The likelihood of pelvic involvement is also related to the number of positive inguinal lymph nodes and also the presence of extranodal extension in the inguinal specimen.[2,38] Recently, Lughezzani and colleagues[39] suggested the diameter of metastasis as a predictive factor for pelvic lymph node involvement. Imaging in patients at high risk for pelvic metastasis may show pelvic lymphadenopathy, while assessment of the pelvic lymph nodes in the absence of inguinal nodal involvement is not indicated. Currently CT scanning is not very accurate in predicting pelvic nodal involvement and has a sensitivity of only 20%.[40] However, morphologically suspicious pelvic lymph nodes (defined as short-axis diameter >10 mm and/or central necrosis) in the presence[33] of inguinal nodal involvement are malignant unless proven otherwise.[40] Patients at high risk for pelvic metastasis may benefit from preoperative PET/CT scanning.[41] Although no direct comparison has been made between PET/CT scanning and CT imaging, PET/CT scanning is likely to be more accurate in the preoperative staging of the pelvic lymph nodes. This is primarily based upon the experience in other malignancies.[32–34] Additionally, distant metastasis can be identified with PET/CT scanning due to whole-body scanning. The use of other imaging modalities (eg, MRI) to stage the pelvic lymph nodes in patients with penile carcinoma has not been fully evaluated.[41]

MINIMALLY INVASIVE STAGING TECHNIQUES

To circumvent the previously mentioned dilemmas regarding lymphadenectomy, minimally invasive staging techniques have been developed. The basis of these techniques is to limit the morbidity in patients with pathological node-negative groins, and to identify occult metastases at the earliest opportunity. Only patients with proven lymphatic spread undergo a completion therapeutic radical lymphadenectomy. In the last 2 decades, 2 approaches have been introduced worldwide: modified inguinal lymphadenectomy (MIL) and dynamic sentinel node biopsy (DSNB).

MODIFIED INGUINAL LYMPHADENECTOMY

MIL was proposed by Catalona in 1988 after being performed in 6 patients with invasive carcinoma of the penis or distal urethra. The aim of this approach is to remove the lymph nodes at the most probable location of first-line lymphatic invasion. The anatomic boundaries are the adductor longus muscle, the lateral border of the femoral artery, the inguinal ligament with the inferior margin, and the fascia lata just distal to the fossa ovalis. The lymph node package can be analyzed by frozen section, and if it confirms metastatic disease, then a radical inguinal lymphadenectomy can be performed. The advantage of this MIL is a smaller skin incision and a smaller node dissection, resulting in reduced morbidity compared with standard radical lymphadenectomy. However, limiting the dissection field has led to a high number of false-negative findings as reported by several other authors.

Several case studies have attested to this unreliability with nodal recurrences after negative MIL varying from 0% to 15%. To date there is no information regarding the morbidity of the procedure. The claims of its low morbidity are not substantiated so far, as no direct comparison has been made to radical lymphadenectomy.

SENTINEL NODE BIOPSY

Sentinel node biopsy for penile cancer was first reported by Cabañas in 1977. This was based on lymphangiograms of the penis, and the lymph node medial to the superficial epigastric vein was identified as being the first echelon lymph node or so-called sentinel node. It was assumed that a negative sentinel node was indicative for absence of further lymphatic spread, and therefore no lymphadenectomy was indicated. Sentinel node surgery consisted of identification and removal of this lymph node with completion lymphadenectomy only in those with a tumor-positive lymph node (**Figs. 1** and **2**). However, this initial static procedure, based on anatomic landmarks only, did not take into account individual drainage patterns. Several false-negative results were reported, and the technique was largely abandoned. The sentinel node procedure was revived by Morton and colleagues in 1992, by using patent blue-V or isosulfan blue dye as a tracer enabling individual lymphatic mapping. This technique, with the addition of a preoperative radioactive tracer (technetium-99m-labeled nanocolloid ^{99m}Tc), forms the basis of the

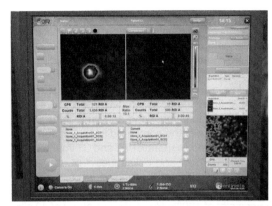

Fig. 2. Screen image of the mobile PET camera before (*left screen*) and after removal (*right screen*) of the SN.

modern sentinel node biopsy era and is also used in breast cancer and melanoma.

Since 1994, DSNB has been performed at the Netherlands Cancer Institute to stage clinically node-negative patients, and in those patients, the 5-year survival has improved significantly.

TECHNIQUE OF DYNAMIC SENTINEL NODE BIOPSY

Conventional lymphoscintigraphy is performed following the injection of ^{99m}Tc nanocolloid intradermally just proximal to the tumor or coronal sulcus. Care has to be taken to encompass the whole tumor region. Once localized, the sentinel nodes are marked on the skin. Intraoperatively, the penis is injected with patent blue dye (Blue Patenté V, Laboratoire Guerbet, Aulnay-Sous-Bois, France). A gamma-ray detection probe and/or gamma-ray camera (Sentinella, OncoVision, Valencia, Spain) is then used to identify and remove the radioactive lymph nodes that directly drain the penis as identified by the lymphoscintigraphy1-10 (**Figs. 3–5**). Patients who are found to have tumor within the sentinel lymph

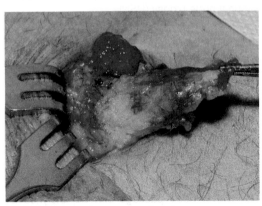

Fig. 1. Removal of the sentinel node.

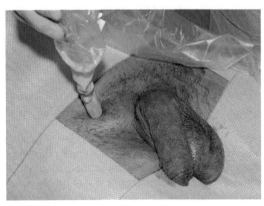

Fig. 3. Gamma-ray detection probe.

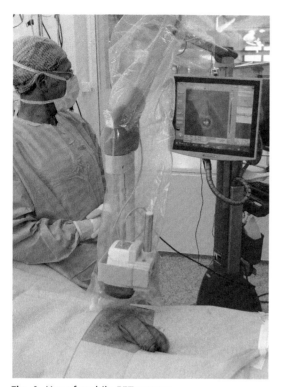

Fig. 4. Use of mobile PET-camera.

nodes undergo a completion lymphadenectomy. Compared with the previously mentioned static procedure first described by Cabañas, the dynamic approach visualizes the individual drainage patterns for each individual patient.

The DSNB procedure for penis cancer was first described in 2001. With this dynamic approach, an initial sensitivity of 80% was reported. In the following years, the DSNB protocol has been modified after detailed analysis of the false-negative cases. The initial procedure was extended by pathologic examination of the sentinel node by serial sectioning and immunohistochemical staining instead of routine paraffin sections, and addition of preoperative ultrasonography with FNAC to detect pathologically enlarged nodes that fail to detect radioactivity. Furthermore, exploration of groins with nonvisualization on preoperative lymphoscintigram (occurring in approximately 4%–20% of clinically node-negative groins) and intraoperative palpation of the wound has been introduced. The modified procedure has evolved into a reliable minimally invasive staging technique with an associated sensitivity of 85% to 95% together with a low morbidity.

More recently, fluorescence has been introduced to the diagnostic procedure, and a fluorescent or hybrid (radioactive and fluorescent) tracer is used: indocyanine green (ICG) either or not paired with (99m)Tc-nanocolloid (**Figs. 6** and **7**). This hybrid tracer follows the same drainage pattern as the standard radioactive-only tracer, and the use of it has significantly improved intraoperative optical visualization of sentinel nodes in a study of 65 patients (it enabled visualization of 96.8% of sentinel nodes when 55.7% was blue only).

The latest development in the DSNB procedure is a 3-dimensional reconstruction based on preoperative single-photon emission computed tomography (SPECT)/CT, enabling per-operative navigation. Because a reference device is placed on the patient during SPECT/CT and operation, navigation in the 3-dimensional model is possible intraoperatively (**Figs. 8** and **9**).

SETTINGS FOR DYNAMIC SENTINEL NODE BIOPSY

DSNB is a versatile tool that can be used in several clinical settings:

Bilateral clinically node-negative patients
Unilateral clinically node-negative patients, while the other node-positive side is managed by a formal lymphadenectomy

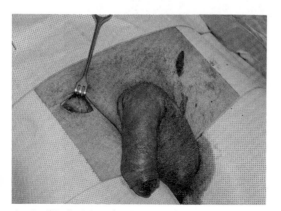

Fig. 5. Skin incisions for SN procedure.

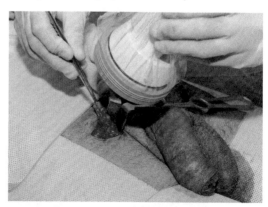

Fig. 6. Use of near infrared camera for fluorescence detection.

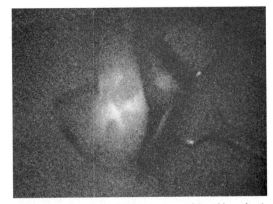

Fig. 7. Screen image of fluorescent node and lymphatic channels.

Unilateral or bilateral clinically node-negative patients after the primary tumor has been resected (postresection DSNB)

A second DSNB after initial tumor-negative DSNB in patients who developed a recurrence of a primary tumor

Graafland and colleagues described 12 patients in whom a second DSNB was performed due to penile cancer recurrence. A new sentinel node was identified in 80% of these patients. Other series reported clinically node-negative penile carcinoma after previous therapeutic primary tumor resection. Results were similar to the favorable experience with the DSNB in patients with their tumor still present.

RELIABILITY

In a large prospective series of 323 patients from 2 tertiary referral hospitals that use essentially the same protocol, DSNB was shown to be a reliable method with a low complication rate. The combined sensitivity of this procedure was 93% with a specificity of 100%. Complications occurred in less than 5% of explored groins, and almost all were transient and could be managed conservatively. Some critics of the technique have pointed out that there is an associated learning curve, as the false-negative rate diminished during the years from 20% to 22% initially to a recent 5% to 7%. This is supported by Jakobsen and colleagues, having 50% of their false-negative sentinel node biopsies in the first 30 of 409 groins (first 7%). However, in the previously mentioned series from 2 hospitals, no learning curve could be demonstrated in the initial 30 procedures done at 1 of the 2 hospitals.

STAGING RECOMMENDATIONS

Currently, DSNB is recommended in clinically node-negative groins of patients with penile tumors of at least T1G2. Only patients with a tumor-positive sentinel lymph node should undergo a therapeutic ipsilateral inguinal lymphadenectomy. Compliant patients with lower-risk tumors (pTis, pTa, and pT1G1) can be managed with close surveillance followed by lymphadenectomy if metastases become clinically apparent.

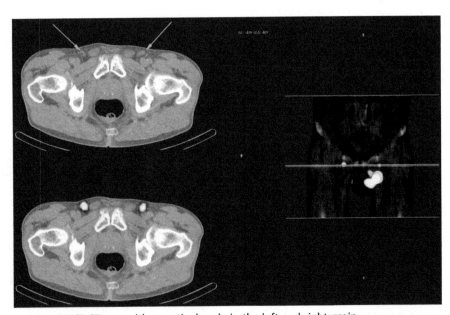

Fig. 8. Preoperative SPECT-CT scan with a sentinel node in the left and right groin.

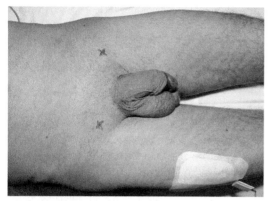

Fig. 9. Preoperative skin markings.

REFERENCES

1. Horenblas S, van Tinteren H. Squamous cell carcinoma of the penis. IV. Prognostic factors of survival: analysis of tumor, nodes and metastasis classification system. J Urol 1994;151(5):1239–43.
2. Lont AP, Kroon BK, Gallee MP, et al. Pelvic lymph node dissection for penile carcinoma: extent of inguinal lymph node involvement as an indicator for pelvic lymph node involvement and survival. J Urol 2007;177(3):947–52 [discussion: 52].
3. Sanchez-Ortiz RF, Pettaway CA. The role of lymphadenectomy in penile cancer. Urol Oncol 2004;22(3): 236–44 [discussion: 44–5].
4. Pandey D, Mahajan V, Kannan RR. Prognostic factors in node-positive carcinoma of the penis. J Surg Oncol 2006;93(2):133–8.
5. Ornellas AA, Nobrega BL, Wei Kin Chin E, et al. Prognostic factors in invasive squamous cell carcinoma of the penis: analysis of 196 patients treated at the Brazilian National Cancer Institute. J Urol 2008;180(4):1354–9.
6. Sun M, Djajadiningrat RS, Alnajjar HM, et al. Development and external validation of a prognostic tool for prediction of cancer-specific mortality after complete loco-regional pathological staging for squamous cell carcinoma of the penis. BJU Int 2015;116(5):734–43.
7. Djajadiningrat RS, Graafland NM, van Werkhoven E, et al. Contemporary management of regional nodes in penile cancer—improvement of survival? J Urol 2014;191(1):68–73.
8. Srinivas V, Morse MJ, Herr HW, et al. Penile cancer: relation of extent of nodal metastasis to survival. J Urol 1987;137(5):880–2.
9. Wespes E. The management of regional lymph nodes in patients with penile carcinoma and reliability of sentinel node biopsy. Eur Urol 2007;52(1):15–6 [discussion: 20–1].
10. Solsona E, Algaba F, Horenblas S, et al, European Association of Urology. EAU guidelines on penile cancer. Eur Urol 2004;46(1):1–8.
11. Hegarty PK, Kayes O, Freeman A, et al. A prospective study of 100 cases of penile cancer managed according to European Association of Urology guidelines. BJU Int 2006;98(3):526–31.
12. Ercole CE, Pow-Sang JM, Spiess PE. Update in the surgical principles and therapeutic outcomes of inguinal lymph node dissection for penile cancer. Urol Oncol 2013;31(5):505–16.
13. Ravi R. Morbidity following groin dissection for penile carcinoma. Br J Urol 1993;72(6):941–5.
14. Ornellas AA, Seixas AL, de Moraes JR. Analyses of 200 lymphadenectomies in patients with penile carcinoma. J Urol 1991;146(2):330–2.
15. Bevan-Thomas R, Slaton JW, Pettaway CA. Contemporary morbidity from lymphadenectomy for penile squamous cell carcinoma: the M.D. Anderson Cancer Center experience. J Urol 2002; 167(4):1638–42.
16. Stuiver MM, Djajadiningrat RS, Graafland NM, et al. Early wound complications after inguinal lymphadenectomy in penile cancer: a historical cohort study and risk-factor analysis. Eur Urol 2013;64(3):486–92.
17. McDougal WS. Carcinoma of the penis: improved survival by early regional lymphadenectomy based on the histological grade and depth of invasion of the primary lesion. J Urol 1995;154(4):1364–6.
18. Lont AP, Horenblas S, Tanis PJ, et al. Management of clinically node negative penile carcinoma: improved survival after the introduction of dynamic sentinel node biopsy. J Urol 2003;170(3):783–6.
19. Kroon BK, Horenblas S, Lont AP, et al. Patients with penile carcinoma benefit from immediate resection of clinically occult lymph node metastases. J Urol 2005;173(3):816–9.
20. Persson B, Sjodin JG, Holmberg L, et al. The National Penile Cancer Register in Sweden 2000–2003. Scand J Urol Nephrol 2007;41(4):278–82.
21. Ornellas AA, Seixas AL, Marota A, et al. Surgical treatment of invasive squamous cell carcinoma of the penis: retrospective analysis of 350 cases. J Urol 1994;151(5):1244–9.
22. Djajadiningrat RS, Teertstra HJ, van Werkhoven E, et al. Ultrasound examination and fine needle aspiration cytology-useful for followup of the regional nodes in penile cancer? J Urol 2014;191(3):652–5.
23. Ornellas AA, Kinchin EW, Nobrega BL, et al. Surgical treatment of invasive squamous cell carcinoma of the penis: Brazilian National Cancer Institute long-term experience. J Surg Oncol 2008;97(6): 487–95.
24. Kirrander P, Sherif A, Friedrich B, et al, Steering Committee of the Swedish National Penile Cancer Register. Swedish National Penile Cancer Register: incidence, tumour characteristics, management and survival. BJU Int 2016;117(2):287–92.
25. Kroon BK, Horenblas S, Deurloo EE, et al. Ultrasonography-guided fine-needle aspiration cytology

before sentinel node biopsy in patients with penile carcinoma. BJU Int 2005;95(4):517–21.

26. Saisorn I, Lawrentschuk N, Leewansangtong S, et al. Fine-needle aspiration cytology predicts inguinal lymph node metastasis without antibiotic pretreatment in penile carcinoma. BJU Int 2006; 97(6):1225–8.

27. Horenblas S, Van Tinteren H, Delemarre JF, et al. Squamous cell carcinoma of the penis: accuracy of tumor, nodes and metastasis classification system, and role of lymphangiography, computerized tomography scan and fine needle aspiration cytology. J Urol 1991;146(5):1279–83.

28. Jensen JB, Jensen KM, Ulhoi BP, et al. Sentinel lymph-node biopsy in patients with squamous cell carcinoma of the penis. BJU Int 2009;103(9): 1199–203.

29. Graafland NM, Teertstra HJ, Besnard AP, et al. Identification of high risk pathological node positive penile carcinoma: value of preoperative computerized tomography imaging. J Urol 2011;185(3): 881–7.

30. Tabatabaei S, Harisinghani M, McDougal WS. Regional lymph node staging using lymphotropic nanoparticle enhanced magnetic resonance imaging with ferumoxtran-10 in patients with penile cancer. J Urol 2005;174(3):923–7 [discussion: 7].

31. Thoeny HC, Triantafyllou M, Birkhaeuser FD, et al. Combined ultrasmall superparamagnetic particles of iron oxide-enhanced and diffusion-weighted magnetic resonance imaging reliably detect pelvic lymph node metastases in normal-sized nodes of bladder and prostate cancer patients. Eur Urol 2009;55(4):761–9.

32. Lardinois D, Weder W, Hany TF, et al. Staging of non-small-cell lung cancer with integrated positron-emission tomography and computed tomography. N Engl J Med 2003;348(25):2500–7.

33. Antoch G, Saoudi N, Kuehl H, et al. Accuracy of whole-body dual-modality fluorine-18-2-fluoro-2-deoxy-D-glucose positron emission tomography and computed tomography (FDG-PET/CT) for tumor staging in solid tumors: comparison with CT and PET. J Clin Oncol 2004;22(21):4357–68.

34. Ng SH, Yen TC, Chang JT, et al. Prospective study of [18F]fluorodeoxyglucose positron emission tomography and computed tomography and magnetic resonance imaging in oral cavity squamous cell carcinoma with palpably negative neck. J Clin Oncol 2006;24(27):4371–6.

35. Scher B, Seitz M, Reiser M, et al. 18F-FDG PET/CT for staging of penile cancer. J Nucl Med 2005; 46(9):1460–5.

36. Leijte JA, Graafland NM, Valdes Olmos RA, et al. Prospective evaluation of hybrid 18F-fluorodeoxyglucose positron emission tomography/computed tomography in staging clinically node-negative patients with penile carcinoma. BJU Int 2009;104(5): 640–4.

37. Sadeghi R, Gholami H, Zakavi SR, et al. Accuracy of 18F-FDG PET/CT for diagnosing inguinal lymph node involvement in penile squamous cell carcinoma: systematic review and meta-analysis of the literature. Clin Nucl Med 2012;37(5):436–41.

38. Zhu Y, Zhang SL, Ye DW, et al. Prospectively packaged ilioinguinal lymphadenectomy for penile cancer: the disseminative pattern of lymph node metastasis. J Urol 2009;181(5):2103–8.

39. Lughezzani G, Catanzaro M, Torelli T, et al. The relationship between characteristics of inguinal lymph nodes and pelvic lymph node involvement in penile squamous cell carcinoma: a single institution experience. J Urol 2014;191(4):977–82.

40. Zhu Y, Zhang SL, Ye DW, et al. Predicting pelvic lymph node metastases in penile cancer patients: a comparison of computed tomography, Cloquet's node, and disease burden of inguinal lymph nodes. Onkologie 2008;31(1–2):37–41.

41. Graafland NM, Leijte JA, Valdes Olmos RA, et al. Scanning with 18F-FDG-PET/CT for detection of pelvic nodal involvement in inguinal node-positive penile carcinoma. Eur Urol 2009;56(2):339–45.

Surgical Advances in Inguinal Lymph Node Dissection
Optimizing Treatment Outcomes

Pranav Sharma, MD[a], Homayoun Zargar, MBChB, FRACS(Urol)[b,c],
Philippe E. Spiess, MD, MS, FRCS(C)[a,*]

KEYWORDS

- Penile cancer • Inguinal lymph node dissection • Pelvic lymph node dissection • Surgery • Survival
- Complications

KEY POINTS

- Antibiotic treatment before inguinal lymph node dissection (ILND) in patients with palpable inguinal nodes is not recommended.
- Radical ILND is associated with postoperative complications, including hematoma, lymphocele, or seroma formation, skin necrosis, wound infection or dehiscence, and chronic scrotal or lower extremity edema.
- Modifications to ILND including preservation of the saphenous vein and fascia lata, avoidance of dissection lateral to the femoral artery, and elimination of Sartorius muscle transposition have reduced its perioperative morbidity.
- Video endoscopy ILND (VEIL) or robotic-assisted laparoscopic ILND are minimally invasive options for the treatment of patients with penile cancer offering the potential of fewer complications without compromising oncological outcomes when performed in appropriately selected patients.
- For men with 2 or more positive ILNs or inguinal extracapsular extension (pN3), an ipsilateral or bilateral PLND is indicated for appropriate surgical treatment and staging.

INTRODUCTION

The presence and extent of regional lymph node (LN) metastases is one of the most important prognostic factors in determining the long-term survival of patients with penile cancer.[1] Cure can be achieved in patients with metastatic disease confined to these nodes, so its management is crucial in determining oncological outcomes.[2]

Physical examination of the groin and pelvis, therefore, is an important component of the evaluation of a patient with penile cancer.[3] Evaluation of the inguinal LNs (ILNs) should assess and describe the presence and palpability of enlarged nodes or masses in the groin, the number of LNs present, their size (ie, diameter or dimensions), unilateral versus bilateral localization, the mobility or fixation of inguinal nodes or masses, their relationship to other adjacent structures (ie, Cooper ligament) and/or involvement of the overlying skin, and the presence or absence of edema of the penis, scrotum, and/or legs.

The authors wish to confirm that there are no known conflicts of interest associated with this publication and there has been no significant financial support for this work that could have influenced its outcome.

[a] Department of Genitourinary Oncology, H. Lee Moffitt Cancer Center, 12902 Magnolia Drive, Tampa, FL 33612, USA; [b] Australian Prostate Cancer Research Centre, Melbourne, Victoria 3051, Australia; [c] Department of Urology, Royal Melbourne Hospital, Melbourne, Victoria 3051, Australia
* Corresponding author.
E-mail address: philippe.spiess@moffitt.org

urologic.theclinics.com

The presence of pelvic or retroperitoneal LNs, as well as distant metastatic disease also needs to be assessed with cross-sectional imaging (ie, computed tomography [CT] or MRI).[4]

18F-fluorodeoxyglucose (FDG) PET-CT has recently come to the forefront in the staging of penile cancer due to its increased utilization with other malignant diseases.[5] Studies show that this imaging modality may be useful in confirming inguinal and pelvic metastatic spread, although its ability to detect micro-metastasis has come into question due to higher false-negative rates.[6–8] A comprehensive systematic review and meta-analysis of the literature reported a pooled sensitivity of 96.4% for cN+ patients and 56.5% for cN0 patients for 18F-FDG PET-CT in the accuracy of predicting ILN invasion for penile squamous cell carcinoma (SCC).[9] The investigators, therefore, concluded that routine use of PET-CT was not justified, but patients with clinically palpable ILNs may benefit from additional imaging to confirm presence of disease. Larger prospective clinical trials, however, comparing PET-CT to standard clinical assessment are necessary to determine the true benefits that this technology can provide.

Lymphatic drainage from the primary penile tumor follows a predictable pattern.[10,11] The superficial ILNs located between Scarpa fascia and the fascia lata are the first regional nodal packet affected by metastatic lymphatic spread with up to 25 LNs found in this zone of dissection. The most common site of initial metastasis to the superficial ILNs is the superomedial zone (**Fig. 1**).[12] Lymphatic drainage is rarely seen directly from the primary penile tumor to the inferior regions of the groin based on anatomic imaging studies.[13]

The second regional nodal packet affected by metastatic lymphatic spread is the deep ILNs located beneath the fascia lata and medial to the femoral vein with up to 5 LNs found in this zone of dissection.[14] The femoral artery and nerve are also located in this region, so care must be taken during lymphadenectomy to avoid major vascular or nerve-related injuries.

Metastatic lymphatic spread can be unilateral or bilateral to the groins from the primary penile tumor.[11] Lymphatic drainage is bilateral in 80% of patients with penile cancer, unilateral in 18% of cases, and no drainage is seen in 2% of patients with penile cancer.[15] Crossover metastatic lymphatic spread from right to left groin or left to right groin also can occur.

After inguinal metastatic lymphatic spread, the pelvic LNs, including the obturator, external iliac, and internal iliac LNs are the next regional nodal packets affected by disease dissemination.[10] Direct lymphatic drainage from the primary penile

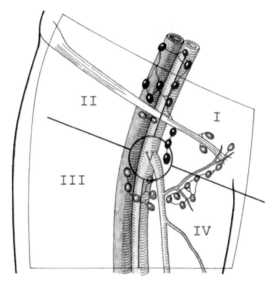

Fig. 1. Lymphatic drainage of penile cancer to the superficial inguinal lymph nodes; the region is divided into 5 zones: superomedial (I), superolateral (II), inferolateral (III), inferomedial (IV), and central (V). (*From* Protzel C, Alcaraz A, Horenblas S, et al. Lymphadenectomy in the surgical management of penile cancer. Eur Urol 2009;55(5):1075–88; with permission.)

tumor to the pelvic LNs, however, has never been described (ie, skip lesions) and metastatic lymphatic spread from the groin to the contralateral pelvic LNs has never been reported in patients with penile cancer. Additionally, the occurrence of crossover metastatic lymphatic spread from the right to left pelvis or left to right pelvis has never been demonstrated. Pelvic nodal disease, therefore, does not seem to occur without ipsilateral ILN disease.[13]

Further spread of penile malignancy from the pelvic LNs to the para-aortic, paracaval, or other retroperitoneal LNs is considered systemic metastatic disease beyond the regional lymphatic drainage system of the penis. This occurs before spread to other visceral organs, including the lungs, liver, and bone.

CLINICAL INDICATIONS FOR LYMPH NODE DISSECTION

For patients with penile cancer with clinically normal groins on physical examination, the risk of inguinal metastatic spread is dependent on the stage, grade, and presence of lymphovascular invasion (LVI) in the primary penile tumor.[16] Low-grade penile lesions (G1/G2) and pTis, pTa, or pT1 tumors without LVI (pT1a) have a low risk of inguinal lymphatic spread.[17] Surveillance, therefore, is recommended for patients with penile cancer in this setting with serial physical examinations and cross-sectional imaging.[18] A prerequisite for surveillance, however, is adequate patient education, understanding, and good patient compliance with follow-up.

High-grade penile lesions (G3/G4), pT1 tumors with LVI (pT1b), and pT2 to pT4 tumors have a 20% to 30% risk of micrometastatic ILN disease even in the presence of clinically normal groins.[19,20] ILN dissection (ILND), therefore, is recommended for patients with penile cancer in this setting because early bilateral ILND results in better 5-year overall survival (OS) compared with radiotherapy or surveillance alone (74% vs 66% vs 63%, respectively).[21] Delaying ILND in intermediate-risk (pT1b disease) or high-risk (G3/G4 or pT2–T4 disease) patients with penile cancer until groins become clinically positive results in worse long-term oncological outcomes.[22] Patient survival is more than 90% with early lymphadenectomy and less than 40% with lymphadenectomy for later regional recurrence.[23]

Kakies and colleagues[24] raised concern with the use of tumor grade as a surrogate indicator for ILND in clinically node-negative patients, as well as its integration into the current TNM classification for penile cancer. The investigators reported a high degree of interobserver variability with the classification of penile carcinomas into various grade categories, and they argued that the low reproducibility of grading in penile cancer does not allow for a reliable prognostication of tumor aggressiveness. Further large-scale studies, however, are necessary to reproduce these findings to provide clarification on the role of tumor grade.

For patients with penile cancer with unilateral (cN1) or bilateral (cN2) clinically palpable ILNs on physical examination, the risk of inguinal lymphatic spread is very high, so ILND is recommended for complete disease staging and treatment.[25] For clinically questionable cases (ie, patients with low-risk primary penile tumors), fine-needle aspiration (FNA) of clinically suspicious nodes under ultrasound guidance with cytology is recommended for an immediate diagnosis rather than 4 to 6 weeks of antibiotic therapy to rule out LN enlargement from infectious or inflammatory processes.[26,27] Antibiotic treatment to exclude LN enlargement due to infection is no longer warranted because oncological diagnosis and treatment should be undertaken without delay before further metastatic spread occurs.[16]

For patients with penile cancer with clinically bulky (>4 cm) palpable ILNs or fixed regional ILN disease, chemotherapy is recommended initially followed by surgical resection with ILND in responsive cases, as nonresponders do poorly with rapid progression to systemic metastatic disease.[28] Additionally, upfront surgery may result in unnecessary surgical morbidity with the requirement for vascular resection and reconstruction or excision of a large amount of skin requiring skin graft or muscle flap closure.[29]

Approximately 20% to 30% of patients with positive ILNs will also have metastatic lymphatic spread to the pelvic LNs (PLNs).[30] Patients with pelvic nodal metastasis have a poor overall prognosis (5-year OS of 10%), especially when compared with patients with only inguinal metastatic disease.[31] Patients who have only 1 positive ILN have a risk of PLN involvement of less than 5%.[32] PLN dissection (PLND), therefore, is recommended for patients with penile cancer with 2 or more positive ILNs or with ILNs with extracapsular extension (ECE) (pN3) found during ILND.[33,34] Prophylactic PLND in these cases may have some curative potential in pelvic node–positive cases with micro-metastatic disease with reported cure rates ranging from 16% to 20%.[35]

PLND can be done during the same operative setting (with use of intraoperative frozen section) or in a delayed fashion through an open midline suprapubic extraperitoneal approach.[36] Because no crossover from ILNs to PLNs has been described, the use of unilateral versus bilateral PLND is still considered controversial in clinically indicated settings. There is increasing evidence, however, that bilateral PLND may be appropriate for certain high-risk patients with high-volume inguinal nodal disease and that bilateral PLND may improve survival-related outcomes in this setting.[37,38] For patients with penile cancer with clinically enlarged pelvic LNs on cross-sectional imaging with CT, MRI, or PET-CT, neoadjuvant chemotherapy is recommended followed by postchemotherapy inguinal and pelvic LND in clinical responders.[39]

A summarized algorithm of the clinical indications for lymphadenectomy for penile carcinoma is provided in **Fig. 2**.

RADICAL INGUINAL LYMPH NODE DISSECTION

Radical ILND is recommended for patients with penile cancer with clinically positive inguinal metastatic disease on physical examination. The boundaries of dissection include the inguinal ligament and the spermatic cord superiorly, the adductor longus muscle medially, the Sartorius muscle laterally, and the floor of dissection consists of the pectineus muscle (**Fig. 3**).[40]

A skin incision is made approximately 1 to 2 cm parallel and inferior to the inguinal ligament from

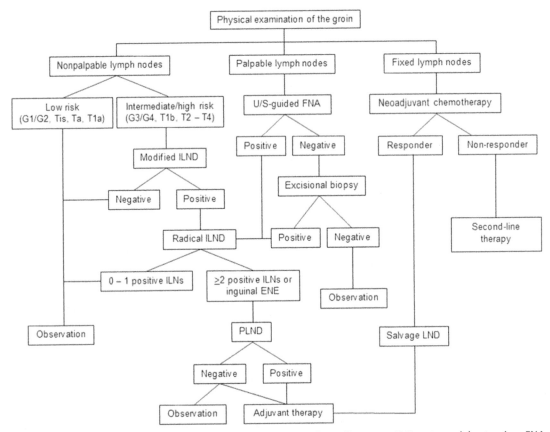

Fig. 2. Flow diagram for the management of ILNs in patients with penile cancer. ENE, extranodal extension; FNA, fine needle aspiration; U/S, ultrasound. (*Adapted from* Protzel C, Alcaraz A, Horenblas S, et al. Lymphadenectomy in the surgical management of penile cancer. Eur Urol 2009;55(5):1075–88; with permission.)

the anterior superior iliac spine laterally to the pubic tubercle medially. When the overlying skin is involved with disease secondary to direct tumor invasion or broken down by infection or prior therapy, an elliptical incision with resection of the skin and the subcutaneous tissue should be considered.[41] The skin edges should be handled gently and care should be taken to preserve the

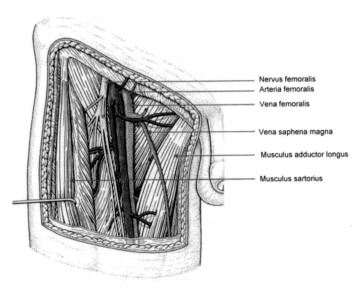

Nervus femoralis
Arteria femoralis
Vena femoralis
Vena saphena magna
Musculus adductor longus
Musculus sartorius

Fig. 3. Anatomy of the inguinofemoral region. (*From* Protzel C, Alcaraz A, Horenblas S, et al. Lymphadenectomy in the surgical management of penile cancer. Eur Urol 2009;55(5):1075–88; with permission.)

superficial blood supply to the flaps. Flap edges should be covered with saline-moistened sponges to prevent from drying out, and grasping of the edges with forceps should be avoided as this could crush and devascularize the tissue.

Dissection is initially started from the aponeurosis of the external oblique and spermatic cord down to the inguinal ligament.[42] The superficial ILNs and areolar tissue are then isolated and removed above the fascia lata using clips for careful control of lymphatic vessels. Dissection is carried through the fascia lata overlying the Sartorius muscle laterally and the adductor longus muscle medially. The ipsilateral deep ILNs are then exposed, isolated, and removed. Dissection is performed along the femoral artery and vein down to the femoral canal. The femoral vessels are skeletonized in the femoral triangle, and resection is carried medially to laterally over the femoral vein, artery, and nerve. The cutaneous nerves and branches of the femoral vascular system supplying the overlying subcutaneous tissue are divided for adequate hemostasis, while the motor nerves are preserved. The long saphenous vein is identified in the femoral triangle, and it is ligated at the level of the saphenofemoral junction. Finally, the Sartorius muscle is transposed as a rotational flap once ILND is complete by releasing its attachments from the anterior superior iliac spine so as to provide myocutaneous coverage over the femoral vessels. The muscle and subcutaneous tissues are then reapproximated to obliterate any potential dead space for a postoperative fluid collection, and the skin is closed, leaving a suction drain in place. If the skin edges do not re-approximate easily or if they are nonviable, a split-thickness skin graft is applied instead.

There are data to suggest that the number of LNs removed as well as LN density can serve as prognostic indicators for long-term treatment outcomes.[43] Li and colleagues[44] suggest that disease-specific survival from penile cancer following radical lymphadenectomy can be predicted by both LN count and LN density. Removal of at least 16 ILNs during surgery in patients with pathologically negative nodes was a significant prognostic indicator of better cancer-specific survival (CSS) compared with patients who are pN0 with fewer than 16 ILNs removed. Additionally, patients with pathologically positive nodes with an LN density greater than 16% had a better CSS compared with patients who were pN+ with an LN density less than 16%. Other investigators have suggested a lymph node density of 22% as an appropriate cutoff to predict CSS in patients with penile cancer.[45] Larger prospective validation studies, however, are needed to support these initial findings.

Radical ILND is associated with significant perioperative patient morbidity with overall complication rates as high as 80% and major complication rates as high as 20%.[29] Common postoperative complications include hematoma, lymphocele, or seroma formation; wound infection; skin necrosis; wound dehiscence; and chronic scrotal or lower extremity edema due to disruption of the lymphatic drainage from the genitals and the legs.[46] Contemporary series have reported a 43% incidence of wound infection, 24% incidence of seroma formation, 16% incidence of skin-flap problems (ie, necrosis or wound breakdown), and 5% to 7% incidence of deep vein thrombosis (DVT) and pulmonary embolism (PE).[47,48]

Based on the largest report of complication rates after ILND for SCC of the penis, median number of LNs removed was an independent predictor of major complications. Disease stage, patient age, ILND with Sartorius flap transposition, and surgery before 2008 were also independent predictors of major wound-related infections.[46]

Use of prophylactic intravenous antibiotics, placement of a percutaneous closed-suction drain postoperatively, meticulous closure of lymphatic vessels with ligation or clips, and early use of compression stockings, sequential pneumatic compression devices, and inguinal pressure dressings can all be used to minimize postoperative adverse events in patients with penile cancer undergoing LND.[49] Prophylactic anticoagulation with low-molecular-weight heparin can also decrease the risk of postoperative DVT or PE.[50]

MODIFIED INGUINAL LYMPH NODE DISSECTION

A modified, limited ILND has been described in an attempt to minimize the postoperative patient morbidity of the surgery.[51] This reported technique includes revisions to minimize postoperative complications, including a shorter skin incision, limiting the area of dissection to the superomedial quadrant of the inguinal region, preservation of the saphenous vein, avoidance of dissection lateral to the femoral artery and caudal to the fossa ovalis, preservation of the fascia lata, and elimination of the Sartorius muscle transposition.[52,53]

This revised technique preserves the superficial blood supply to the skin flaps of the incision, minimizing the risk of postoperative skin necrosis, wound infection, and wound dehiscence with complete incisional breakdown.[54] It also minimizes disturbances to the regional lymphatic drainage system of the lower extremities, reducing the risk of postoperative lymphocele formation and chronic scrotal or lower extremity lymphedema. Conversion to a radical ILND, however, is required in the presence of positive inguinal metastatic disease on frozen section with complete removal of all superficial and deep ILNs, as the true false-negative rate for modified ILND has not been established.[55]

SALVAGE INGUINAL LYMPH NODE DISSECTION

Median time to inguinal recurrence after treatment of the primary penile tumor is approximately 6 months.[56] Salvage ILND may be considered for delayed (>1 year after treatment of the primary penile tumor) inguinal recurrence of penile cancer. Some investigators have suggested that neoadjuvant systemic chemotherapy followed by salvage ILND for locally recurrent inguinal disease can be performed with curative potential.[40]

The boundaries of dissection for salvage ILND are similar to radical ILND with resection outside of the standard template if there is inguinal recurrence outside of the region. It may be a potentially curative treatment option for patients with the development of delayed ILN enlargement in the absence of occult distant metastatic disease with durable long-term survival, especially because the role of chemotherapy or radiation is not well defined in this setting.[57] Postoperative complication rates, however, remain high, with as many as 50% of patients experiencing severe, debilitating lymphedema or significant wound complications, and median OS, nevertheless, remains less than 2 years.

Use of presurgical PET-CT, therefore, may be beneficial in appropriately selecting patients for this highly morbid but potentially curative option, and use of neoadjuvant chemotherapy in this setting could also help identify patients who are likely to experience disease progression after surgery.

SKIN AND SOFT TISSUE COVERAGE AFTER INGUINAL LYMPH NODE DISSECTION

For advanced local disease with skin invasion, after radiation therapy, or with salvage surgery for inguinal disease recurrence, there may be lack of soft tissue or skin coverage, especially in the setting of a compromised initial Sartorius flap. For example, in the presence of fixed ILNs (cN3) with involvement of the overlying Scarpa fascia or skin, wide local excision of the superficial tissue is necessary for appropriate oncological control.[41] Additionally, in salvage procedures following prior inguinal surgery or radiation therapy, there may be the presence of wound breakdown and flap necrosis after a primary closure. A rectus abdominis myocutaneous (RAM) flap, therefore, may be an alternative option to provide appropriate wound coverage in these cases of ILND (**Fig. 4**).[58]

The rectus abdominis muscle is a thin, flat muscle with an independent, dual blood supply.[59] The lower half is supplied by the inferior epigastric artery, whereas the upper half is supplied by the

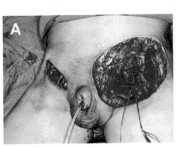
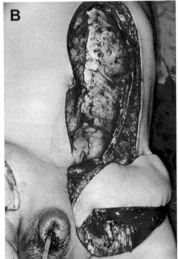
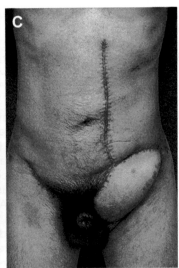

Fig. 4. Utilization of the rectus abdominis flap for groin coverage during salvage ILND (*A–C*). (*From* Aslim EJ, Rasheed MZ, Lin F, et al. Use of the anterolateral thigh and vertical rectus abdominis musculocutaneous flaps as utility flaps in reconstructing large groin defects. Arch Plast Surg 2014;41(5):556–61; with permission.)

superior epigastric artery. The overlying fascia and skin of the RAM flap are supplied by perforating branches of both arteries. This extensive vascular tree is ideally suited for groin coverage with great ease and versatility. Other advantages of the RAM flap include adequate mass to obliterate any potential dead space, ease of donor site closure, and excess skin to allow for a tension-free repair of the inguinal defect.[60] An inferior, epigastric-based vertical or transverse RAM flap can, therefore, provide adequate coverage in the groin for defects as large as 20 cm.

For a RAM flap, the recipient site is prepared after meticulous hemostasis and debridement of all nonviable tissue.[61] Following ILND, the inguinal wound is measured, and an appropriately sized flap is marked on the skin overlying the ipsilateral or contralateral rectus abdominis muscle.

Skin incisions are made in the superior, medial, and lateral aspect of the planned RAM flap, and the underlying subcutaneous tissue, anterior rectus sheath fascia, and rectus abdominis muscle are isolated.[62] The plane between the rectus abdominis muscle and the posterior rectus sheath is then developed to the level of the arcuate line. Subsequently, the inferior epigastric artery is identified and based on this artery, the RAM flap is mobilized by incising the remaining lower portion of the skin and subcutaneous tissue of the flap.

The distal attachments of the rectus abdominis muscle to the pubic bone may sometimes be incised to allow for additional mobility of the flap. Doppler ultrasound also may be used to ensure adequate blood supply from the pedicle of the RAM flap.[63,64] Last, the island of skin and subcutaneous tissue between the base of the flap and the recipient site is incised to the level of the external oblique aponeurosis. The apical portion of the flap is then tunneled to the groin defect and secured appropriately.

MINIMALLY INVASIVE LYMPH NODE DISSECTION

Video endoscopy ILND (VEIL) and robotic-assisted laparoscopy ILND may be used in the future treatment of locally advanced penile cancer with the possibility for reduced postoperative complications and patient morbidity without compromising oncological control and long-term survival-related outcomes. The same surgical and oncological principles of traditional open surgery, however, should be followed with minimally invasive platforms.[65]

The boundaries of surgical dissection are similar to the open approach with the inguinal ligament and spermatic cord located superiorly, the adductor longus muscle medially, and the Sartorius muscle laterally.[66] The saphenous vein may or may not be preserved depending on the degree of surgical exposure necessary to complete the ILND appropriately.

Ideally suited candidates for minimally invasive ILND should include patients with penile cancer with clinically normal groins and nonpalpable ILNs who have high-risk primary penile tumors (ie, pT1b–T4, G3/G4, presence of LVI).[67] Tobias-Machado and colleagues[66] initially reported favorable oncological and cosmetic outcomes with VEIL in a group of patients with clinically negative groins on physical examination. A similar number of ILNs were excised with VEIL compared with standard open ILND, and no reported cases of disease recurrence or progression were noted during follow-up in either group. Overall complication rates were also reduced with VEIL compared with the traditional open approach (20% vs 70%) with less wound-related complications noted with the use of smaller incisions and laparoscopy.[68]

The adoption of minimally invasive robotic-assisted surgery can additionally allow for greater precision and dexterity than standard laparoscopic instruments due to the 3-dimensional optics and improved magnification of the technology.[69] Josephson and colleagues[70] and Sotelo and colleagues[71] both retrospectively reported their experience with robotic-assisted video-endoscopic ILND (RAVEIL) in patients with palpable and nonpalpable ILNs. RAVEIL has also shown the ability to adequately stage inguinal metastatic disease in patients with penile cancer based on a phase 1 prospective study of 10 patients with clinical T1-T3N0 penile carcinoma.[72] Larger, prospective studies with longer-term follow-up, however, are necessary to validate these endoscopic surgical approaches as an alternative treatment option to standard open surgery with similar recurrence patterns and equivalent oncological outcomes.[73]

PELVIC LYMPH NODE DISSECTION

The boundaries of PLND include the bifurcation of the common iliac vessels superiorly, the ilioinguinal nerve laterally, and the obturator nerve medially (**Fig. 5**).[35,38] During PLND, all nodal tissue is removed from the obturator, internal iliac, and external iliac packets, and any clinically enlarged LNs in the pelvis are also removed. Careful control of lymphatic channels with clips or surgical ligation is necessary to prevent development of a postoperative pelvic lymphocele, and appropriate hemostasis should be obtained to prevent excess venous bleeding and a pelvic hematoma.[36]

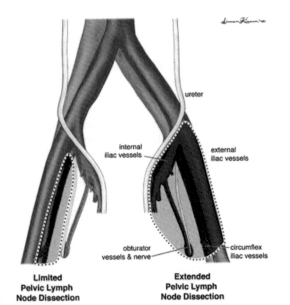

internal
iliac vessels

external
iliac vessels

ureter

obturator
vessels & nerve

circumflex
iliac vessels

Limited Pelvic Lymph Node Dissection

Extended Pelvic Lymph Node Dissection

Fig. 5. Template for PLND. (*From* Yuh B, Artibani W, Heidenreich A, et al. The role of robot-assisted radical prostatectomy and pelvic lymph node dissection in the management of high-risk prostate cancer: a systematic review. Eur Urol 2014;65(5):918–27. [Systematic review/meta-analysis]; with permission.)

SURVEILLANCE STRATEGIES FOLLOWING LYMPHADENECTOMY

Extranodal extension, number of tumor-positive nodes, and pelvic involvement in node-positive (pN+) cases are typically associated with worse 5-year CSS from penile carcinoma, and surveillance strategies following ILND and/or PLND have been constructed taking into account these important prognostic factors (**Table 1**).[74]

Early detection of local recurrence during follow-up increases the likelihood of successful curative treatment and does not significantly reduce long-term survival. Local recurrence is easily detected on physical examination by the patient himself or the physician. Patient education is also an essential part of the follow-up, and patients are counseled to visit their physician if any changes are seen.

Local or regional nodal recurrences usually occur within 2 years of primary treatment.[56] These results support an intensive follow-up regimen every 3 to 6 months during the first 2 years with less intensive follow-up after this every 6 to 12 months for at least a period of 5 years. Although late local recurrences may still occur, life-threatening metastases become very unusual after 5 years. Follow-up after 5 years, therefore, may be omitted in motivated patients reliably able to continue to perform regular self-examinations. In patients unlikely or unwilling to carry out a self-examination, long-term follow-up may be necessary.

Patients with penile cancer without metastatic nodal involvement have a recurrence rate of 2%.[56] In patients with negative ILNs, follow-up should include physical examination of the penis and the groins for early detection of local and/or regional recurrence. The use of ultrasound and FNA cytology in suspicious cases can improve the early detection rate of regional recurrence,[75] but additional imaging with CT, MRI, or PET-CT has no proven benefit (except for obese patients, as a physical examination may be challenging).

Patients with metastatic node-positive disease have a recurrence rate of 19%,[56] so imaging of the chest, abdomen, and pelvis with CT, MRI, or PET-CT is recommended at 3-month to 6-month intervals for the first 2 years due to the risk of development of locoregional or distant metastatic disease. This should complement routine

Table 1
Surveillance guidelines for follow-up of inguinal lymph nodes in penile cancer

	Interval of Follow-up		Investigations			
Nodal Staging	**Year 1–2**	**Year 3–5**	**Physical Examination**	**U/S + FNA Cytology**	**CT/MRI/PET-CT of Chest, Abdomen, and Pelvis**	**Minimum Duration of Follow-up**
Clinically negative groins	3–6 mo	6–12 mo	Yes	No	No	5 y
pN0 at initial treatment with LND	3–6 mo	1 y	Yes	Optional	No	5 y
pN+ at initial treatment with LND	3–6 mo	6–12 mo	Yes	Optional	Yes	5 y

Abbreviations: CT, computed tomography; FNA, fine needle aspiration; LND, lymph node dissection; PET-CT, PET-computed tomography; U/S, ultrasound.

physical examination, and these patients may benefit from adjuvant radiation therapy or systemic chemotherapy.

SUMMARY

ILND for locally advanced penile cancer has evolved over the years with the advent of smaller templates for dissection and increased utilization of minimally invasive technology. This has not only reduced unnecessary patient morbidity from overly extensive surgery, but it has also improved our understanding of the natural pathogenesis and prognostic indicators with this disease. Future prospective studies such as the InPACT (International Penile Advanced Cancer Trial) are needed to elucidate the benefits that more advanced imaging and surgical techniques can provide in terms of early detection of occult metastatic disease in the groin or pelvis, minimizing patient morbidity from unnecessary treatments, and possibly improving short-term and long-term outcomes.

REFERENCES

1. Pow-Sang MR, Ferreira U, Pow-Sang JM, et al. Epidemiology and natural history of penile cancer. Urology 2010;76(2 Suppl 1):S2–6.

2. Horenblas S. Lymphadenectomy in penile cancer. Urol Clin North Am 2011;38(4):459–69, vi–vii.

3. Spiess PE, National Comprehensive Cancer Network. New treatment guidelines for penile cancer. J Natl Compr Canc Netw 2013;11(5 Suppl):659–62.

4. Kayes O, Minhas S, Allen C, et al. The role of magnetic resonance imaging in the local staging of penile cancer. Eur Urol 2007;51(5):1313–8 [discussion: 1318–9].

5. Powles T, Murray I, Brock C, et al. Molecular positron emission tomography and PET/CT imaging in urological malignancies. Eur Urol 2007;51(6):1511–20 [discussion: 1520–1].

6. Graafland NM, Leijte JA, Valdes Olmos RA, et al. Scanning with 18F-FDG-PET/CT for detection of pelvic nodal involvement in inguinal node-positive penile carcinoma. Eur Urol 2009;56(2):339–45.

7. Rosevear HM, Williams H, Collins M, et al. Utility of (1)(8)F-FDG PET/CT in identifying penile squamous cell carcinoma metastatic lymph nodes. Urol Oncol 2012;30(5):723–6.

8. Schlenker B, Scher B, Tiling R, et al. Detection of inguinal lymph node involvement in penile squamous cell carcinoma by 18F-fluorodeoxyglucose PET/CT: a prospective single-center study. Urol Oncol 2012;30(1):55–9.

9. Sadeghi R, Gholami H, Zakavi SR, et al. Accuracy of 18F-FDG PET/CT for diagnosing inguinal lymph node involvement in penile squamous cell carcinoma: systematic review and meta-analysis of the literature. Clin Nucl Med 2012;37(5):436–41 [Systematic review/meta-analysis].

10. Kroon BK, Valdes Olmos RA, van Tinteren H, et al. Reproducibility of lymphoscintigraphy for lymphatic mapping in patients with penile carcinoma. J Urol 2005;174(6):2214–7.

11. Leijte JA, Valdes Olmos RA, Nieweg OE, et al. Anatomical mapping of lymphatic drainage in penile carcinoma with SPECT-CT: implications for the extent of inguinal lymph node dissection. Eur Urol 2008;54(4):885–90.

12. Protzel C, Alcaraz A, Horenblas S, et al. Lymphadenectomy in the surgical management of penile cancer. Eur Urol 2009;55(5):1075–88.

13. Wood HM, Angermeier KW. Anatomic considerations of the penis, lymphatic drainage, and biopsy of the sentinel node. Urol Clin North Am 2010;37(3):327–34.

14. Naumann CM, Al-Najar A, Alkatout I, et al. Lymphatic spread in squamous cell carcinoma of the penis is independent of elevated lymph vessel density. BJU Int 2009;103(12):1655–9 [discussion: 1659].

15. Leijte JA, Hughes B, Graafland NM, et al. Two-center evaluation of dynamic sentinel node biopsy for squamous cell carcinoma of the penis. J Clin Oncol 2009;27(20):3325–9.

16. Hakenberg OW, Comperat EM, Minhas S, et al. EAU guidelines on penile cancer: 2014 update. Eur Urol 2015;67(1):142–50.

17. Bleeker MC, Heideman DA, Snijders PJ, et al. Penile cancer: epidemiology, pathogenesis and prevention. World J Urol 2009;27(2):141–50.

18. Theodorescu D, Russo P, Zhang ZF, et al. Outcomes of initial surveillance of invasive squamous cell carcinoma of the penis and negative nodes. J Urol 1996;155(5):1626–31.

19. Graafland NM, Lam W, Leijte JA, et al. Prognostic factors for occult inguinal lymph node involvement in penile carcinoma and assessment of the high-risk EAU subgroup: a two-institution analysis of 342 clinically node-negative patients. Eur Urol 2010;58(5):742–7.

20. Hughes BE, Leijte JA, Kroon BK, et al. Lymph node metastasis in intermediate-risk penile squamous cell cancer: a two-centre experience. Eur Urol 2010;57(4):688–92.

21. Kulkarni JN, Kamat MR. Prophylactic bilateral groin node dissection versus prophylactic radiotherapy and surveillance in patients with N0 and N1-2A carcinoma of the penis. Eur Urol 1994;26(2):123–8.

22. McDougal WS. Preemptive lymphadenectomy markedly improves survival in patients with cancer of the penis who harbor occult metastases. J Urol 2005;173(3):681.

23. Kroon BK, Horenblas S, Lont AP, et al. Patients with penile carcinoma benefit from immediate resection of clinically occult lymph node metastases. J Urol 2005;173(3):816–9.

24. Kakies C, Lopez-Beltran A, Comperat E, et al. Reproducibility of histopathologic tumor grading in penile cancer–results of a European project. Virchows Arch 2014;464(4):453–61.

25. Heyns CF, Fleshner N, Sangar V, et al. Management of the lymph nodes in penile cancer. Urology 2010; 76(2 Suppl 1):S43–57.

26. Naumann CM, van der Horst S, van der Horst C, et al. Reliability of dynamic sentinel node biopsy combined with ultrasound-guided removal of sonographically suspicious lymph nodes as a diagnostic approach in patients with penile cancer with palpable inguinal lymph nodes. Urol Oncol 2015; 33(9):389.e9-14.

27. Saisorn I, Lawrentschuk N, Leewansangtong S, et al. Fine-needle aspiration cytology predicts inguinal lymph node metastasis without antibiotic pretreatment in penile carcinoma. BJU Int 2006; 97(6):1225–8.

28. Bermejo C, Busby JE, Spiess PE, et al. Neoadjuvant chemotherapy followed by aggressive surgical consolidation for metastatic penile squamous cell carcinoma. J Urol 2007;177(4):1335–8.

29. Bouchot O, Rigaud J, Maillet F, et al. Morbidity of inguinal lymphadenectomy for invasive penile carcinoma. Eur Urol 2004;45(6):761–5 [discussion: 765–6].

30. Liu JY, Li YH, Zhang ZL, et al. The risk factors for the presence of pelvic lymph node metastasis in penile squamous cell carcinoma patients with inguinal lymph node dissection. World J Urol 2013;31(6): 1519–24.

31. Lont AP, Kroon BK, Gallee MP, et al. Pelvic lymph node dissection for penile carcinoma: extent of inguinal lymph node involvement as an indicator for pelvic lymph node involvement and survival. J Urol 2007;177(3):947–52 [discussion: 952].

32. Zhu Y, Zhang SL, Ye DW, et al. Predicting pelvic lymph node metastasis in penile cancer patients: a comparison of computed tomography, Cloquet's node, and disease burden of inguinal lymph nodes. Onkologie 2008;31(1–2):37–41.

33. Lughezzani G, Catanzaro M, Torelli T, et al. The relationship between characteristics of inguinal lymph nodes and pelvic lymph node involvement in penile squamous cell carcinoma: a single institution experience. J Urol 2014;191(4):977–82.

34. Wang JY, Zhu Y, Tang SX, et al. Prognostic significance of the degree of extranodal extension in patients with penile carcinoma. Asian J Androl 2014; 16(3):437–41.

35. Djajadiningrat RS, van Werkhoven E, Horenblas S. Prophylactic pelvic lymph node dissection in patients with penile cancer. J Urol 2015;193(6): 1976–80.

36. Nelson BA, Cookson MS, Smith JA Jr, et al. Complications of inguinal and pelvic lymphadenectomy for squamous cell carcinoma of the penis: a contemporary series. J Urol 2004;172(2):494–7.

37. Zargar-Shoshtari K, Djajadiningrat R, Sharma P, et al. Establishing criteria for bilateral pelvic lymph node dissection in the management of penile cancer: lessons learned from an International Multicenter Collaboration. J Urol 2015; 194(3):696–701.

38. Zargar-Shoshtari K, Sharma P, Djajadiningrat R, et al. Extent of pelvic lymph node dissection in penile cancer may impact survival. World J Urol 2016;34(3):353–9.

39. Giannatempo P, Paganoni A, Sangalli L, et al. Survival analyses of adjuvant or neoadjuvant combination of a taxane plus cisplatin and 5-fluorouracil (T-PF) in patients with bulky nodal metastases from squamous cell carcinoma of the penis (PSCC): results of a single high-volume center. Paper presented at: Journal of Clinical Oncology. San Francisco, January 30-February 1, 2014.

40. Horenblas S. Lymphadenectomy for squamous cell carcinoma of the penis. Part 2: the role and technique of lymph node dissection. BJU Int 2001; 88(5):473–83.

41. Kean J, Hough M, Stevenson JH. Skin excision and groin lymphadenectomy: techniques and outcomes. Lymphology 2006;39(3):141–6.

42. Koifman L, Hampl D, Koifman N, et al. Radical open inguinal lymphadenectomy for penile carcinoma: surgical technique, early complications and late outcomes. J Urol 2013;190(6):2086–92.

43. Zhu Y, Gu CY, Ye DW. Population-based assessment of the number of lymph nodes removed in the treatment of penile squamous cell carcinoma. Urol Int 2014;92(2):186–93.

44. Li ZS, Yao K, Chen P, et al. Disease-specific survival after radical lymphadenectomy for penile cancer: prediction by lymph node count and density. Urol Oncol 2014;32(6):893–900.

45. Lughezzani G, Catanzaro M, Torelli T, et al. Relationship between lymph node ratio and cancer-specific survival in a contemporary series of patients with penile cancer and lymph node metastases. BJU Int 2015;116(5):727–33.

46. Gopman JM, Djajadiningrat RS, Baumgarten AS, et al. Predicting postoperative complications of inguinal lymph node dissection for penile cancer in an international multicentre cohort. BJU Int 2015; 116(2):196–201.

47. Bevan-Thomas R, Slaton JW, Pettaway CA. Contemporary morbidity from lymphadenectomy for penile squamous cell carcinoma: the M.D. Anderson Cancer Center Experience. J Urol 2002;167(4):1638–42.

48. Stuiver MM, Djajadiningrat RS, Graafland NM, et al. Early wound complications after inguinal lymphadenectomy in penile cancer: a historical cohort study and risk-factor analysis. Eur Urol 2013;64(3): 486–92.

49. Spiess PE, Hernandez MS, Pettaway CA. Contemporary inguinal lymph node dissection: minimizing complications. World J Urol 2009;27(2):205–12.

50. Spiess PE. Penile cancer: diagnosis and treatment. Berlin (Germany): Springer Science & Business Media; 2013.

51. Catalona WJ. Modified inguinal lymphadenectomy for carcinoma of the penis with preservation of saphenous veins: technique and preliminary results. J Urol 1988;140(2):306–10.

52. Yao K, Tu H, Li YH, et al. Modified technique of radical inguinal lymphadenectomy for penile carcinoma: morbidity and outcome. J Urol 2010;184(2):546–52.

53. Yao K, Zou ZJ, Li ZS, et al. Fascia lata preservation during inguinal lymphadenectomy for penile cancer: rationale and outcome. Urology 2013;82(3):642–7.

54. Jacobellis U. Modified radical inguinal lymphadenectomy for carcinoma of the penis: technique and results. J Urol 2003;169(4):1349–52.

55. Lopes A, Rossi BM, Fonseca FP, et al. Unreliability of modified inguinal lymphadenectomy for clinical staging of penile carcinoma. Cancer 1996;77(10): 2099–102.

56. Leijte JA, Kirrander P, Antonini N, et al. Recurrence patterns of squamous cell carcinoma of the penis: recommendations for follow-up based on a two-centre analysis of 700 patients. Eur Urol 2008; 54(1):161–8.

57. Baumgarten AS, Alhammali E, Hakky TS, et al. Salvage surgical resection for isolated locally recurrent inguinal lymph node metastasis of penile cancer: international study collaboration. J Urol 2014; 192(3):760–4.

58. Aslim EJ, Rasheed MZ, Lin F, et al. Use of the anterolateral thigh and vertical rectus abdominis musculocutaneous flaps as utility flaps in reconstructing large groin defects. Arch Plast Surg 2014;41(5): 556–61.

59. Slavin SA, Goldwyn RM. The midabdominal rectus abdominis myocutaneous flap: review of 236 flaps. Plast Reconstr Surg 1988;81(2):189–99.

60. Sailon AM, Schachar JS, Levine JP. Free transverse rectus abdominis myocutaneous and deep inferior epigastric perforator flaps for breast reconstruction: a systematic review of flap complication rates and donor-site morbidity. Ann Plast Surg 2009;62(5):560–3 [Systematic review/meta-analysis].

61. Kanchwala SK, Bucky LP. Precision transverse rectus abdominis muscle flap breast reconstruction: a reliable technique for efficient preoperative planning. Ann Plast Surg 2008;60(5):521–6.

62. Gutarra F, Asensio JR, Kohan G, et al. Closure of a contained open abdomen using a bipedicled myofascial oblique rectus abdominis flap technique. J Plast Reconstr Aesthet Surg 2009; 62(11):1490–6.

63. Chen JJ, Giese S, Jeffrey RB, et al. Treatment and stabilization of complex wounds involving the pelvic bone, groin, and femur with the inferiorly based rectus abdominis musculocutaneous flap and the use of power color Doppler imaging in preoperative evaluation. Ann Plast Surg 1999; 43(5):494–8.

64. Georgieu N, Watier E, Fadhul S, et al. Value of pulsed color Doppler before transverse rectus abdominis musculocutaneous flap breast reconstruction. 45 cases. Ann Chir Plast Esthet 2000;45(5): 516–21 [in French].

65. Carmignani G. Words of wisdom. Re: Video endoscopic lymphadenectomy: a new minimally invasive procedure for radical management of inguinal nodes in patients with penile squamous cell carcinoma. Eur Urol 2008;53(2):451–2.

66. Tobias-Machado M, Tavares A, Ornellas AA, et al. Video endoscopic inguinal lymphadenectomy: a new minimally invasive procedure for radical management of inguinal nodes in patients with penile squamous cell carcinoma. J Urol 2007;177(3):953–7 [discussion: 958].

67. Pahwa HS, Misra S, Kumar A, et al. Video endoscopic inguinal lymphadenectomy (VEIL)–a prospective critical perioperative assessment of feasibility and morbidity with points of technique in penile carcinoma. World J Surg Oncol 2013; 11:42.

68. Tobias-Machado M, Tavares A, Silva MN, et al. Can video endoscopic inguinal lymphadenectomy achieve a lower morbidity than open lymph node dissection in penile cancer patients? J Endourol 2008;22(8):1687–91.

69. Autorino R, Zargar H, Akca O, et al. Robot-assisted laparoendoscopic single-site inguinal lymphadenectomy: initial investigation in a cadaver model. Minerva Urol Nefrol 2016;68(3):311–4.

70. Josephson DY, Jacobsohn KM, Link BA, et al. Robotic-assisted endoscopic inguinal lymphadenectomy. Urology 2009;73(1):167–70 [discussion: 170–1].

71. Sotelo R, Cabrera M, Carmona O, et al. Robotic bilateral inguinal lymphadenectomy in penile cancer, development of a technique without robot repositioning: a case report. Ecancermedicalscience 2013;7:356.

72. Matin SF, Cormier JN, Ward JF, et al. Phase 1 prospective evaluation of the oncological adequacy of robotic assisted video-endoscopic inguinal lymphadenectomy in patients with penile carcinoma. BJU Int 2013;111(7):1068–74.

73. Kharadjian TB, Matin SF, Pettaway CA. Early experience of robotic-assisted inguinal lymphadenectomy: review of surgical outcomes relative to alternative approaches. Curr Urol Rep 2014; 15(6):412.

74. Djajadiningrat RS, Graafland NM, van Werkhoven E, et al. Contemporary management of regional nodes in penile cancer—improvement of survival? J Urol 2014;191(1):68–73.

75. Djajadiningrat RS, Teertstra HJ, van Werkhoven E, et al. Ultrasound examination and fine needle aspiration cytology—useful for followup of the regional nodes in penile cancer? J Urol 2014; 191(3):652–5.

Multimodal Therapy in the Management of Advanced Penile Cancer

Praful Ravi, MBBChir[a], Lance C. Pagliaro, MD[b],*

KEYWORDS

- Penile cancer • Adjuvant chemotherapy • Neoadjuvant chemotherapy • Survival • Radiotherapy

KEY POINTS

- A multimodal approach to therapy is increasingly used in treating men with advanced penile cancer.
- Adjuvant chemotherapy is associated with improved outcomes in chemotherapy-naïve men with node-positive penile cancer.
- Neoadjuvant systemic chemotherapy may downstage regional lymph node metastases sufficiently to permit surgery while imparting a potential improvement in long-term disease-free survival.
- International collaboration in clinical trials is required to optimize treatment and improve survival in men with advanced penile cancer.

INTRODUCTION

Squamous cell carcinoma (SCC) of the penis is a rare disease, with an estimated 2020 cases and 340 deaths in the United States this year.[1] Prognosis is good if disease is diagnosed at a localized stage, but up to 40% of patients present with locally advanced or metastatic disease and outcomes for these patients have historically been poor.[2,3] The disease typically spreads in a locoregional manner, first to the draining inguinal lymph nodes, then to pelvic nodes, and then to viscera. The organized nature of spread makes the disease a candidate for a multimodal therapeutic approach, which has been successfully used to treat other SCCs, such as head and neck,[4] anus,[5] or vulva.[6] The rarity of penile cancer in the United States and Western Europe, however, has hampered clinical study into the treatment of locally advanced or metastatic disease and there are currently no randomized data in this setting.

The TNM staging system for penile cancer is shown in **Table 1**. Advanced disease implies spread beyond the local tissues (ie, T3-4 and/or N1-3 and/or M1 disease); 28% to 64% of men with penile cancer present with clinically palpable inguinal lymph nodes. In such cases, metastatic disease underlies lymphadenopathy in 47% to 85% of such individuals, with the remainder due to inflammatory nodal reaction, and the risk of pelvic nodal metastases is 22% to 56% if the inguinal nodes are involved.[7–9] The most important prognostic factor in penile cancer is the presence of inguinal lymph node metastases, with the number of positive lymph nodes, bilateral inguinal nodal disease, pelvic nodal involvement, and extranodal metastatic extension imparting a worse prognosis.[10] When inguinal lymphadenopathy is not clinically apparent, micrometastatic disease is present in approximately 25% of cases, with predictive risk factors including tumor stage, grade, and lymphovascular invasion.[11]

ADJUVANT CHEMOTHERAPY IN NODE-POSITIVE DISEASE

A multimodal approach can be used to treat men who are found node-positive after undergoing

The authors declare no conflicts of interest and no funding source.
[a] Department of Internal Medicine, Mayo Clinic, 200 First Street Southwest, Rochester, MN 55905, USA;
[b] Department of Oncology, Mayo Clinic, 200 First Street Southwest, Rochester, MN 55905, USA
* Corresponding author.
E-mail address: pagliaro.lance@mayo.edu

Table 1
TNM staging system for penile cancer

T – primary tumor
  Tx: Cannot be assessed
  T0: No evidence of primary tumor
  Tis: Carcinoma in situ
  Ta: Noninvasive carcinoma
  T1a: Tumor invades subepithelial tissue without LVI and is not poorly differentiated/undifferentiated
  T1b: Tumor invades subepithelial tissue with LVI or is poorly-differentiated/undifferentiated
  T2: Tumor invades corpus spongiosum and/or cavernosum
  T3: Tumor invades urethra
  T4: Tumor invades other adjacent structures
N – regional lymph nodes
  Nx: Cannot be assessed
  N0: No palpable or visibly enlarged inguinal lymph node
  N1: Palpable mobile unilateral inguinal lymph node
  N2: Palpable mobile multiple unilateral or bilateral inguinal lymph nodes
  N3: Fixed inguinal nodal mass or pelvic lymphadenopathy, unilateral or bilateral
M – distant metastasis
  M0: No distant metastasis
  M1: Distant metastasis
Pathologic classification
  pNX: Cannot be assessed
  pN0: No regional lymph node metastasis
  pN1: Metastasis in a single inguinal lymph node
  pN2: Metastasis in multiple or bilateral inguinal lymph nodes
  pN3: Extranodal extension of lymph node metastasis or pelvic lymph node(s) metastasis

Anatomic staging

Stage	T	N	M
Stage 0	Tis	N0	M0
	Ta	N0	M0
Stage I	T1a	N0	M0
Stage II	T1b	N0	M0
	T2	N0	M0
	T3	N0	M0
Stage IIIA	T1-3	N1	M0
Stage IIIB	T1-3	N2	M0
Stage IV	T4	Any N	M0
	Any T	N3	M0
	Any T	Any N	M1

Abbreviation: LVI, lymphovascular invasion.
Adapted from Sobin LH, Gospodariwicz M, Wittekind C, editors. TNM classification of malignant tumors. UICC International Union Against Cancer. 7th edition. Oxford: Wiley-Blackwell; 2009. p. 336.

radical inguinal lymphadenectomy. Although there is evidence to support the use of adjuvant chemotherapy in men with pN2 or pN3 disease, this is based on small numbers of patients and single-center or multicenter retrospective data.

The largest patient series reporting outcomes of adjuvant chemotherapy for penile cancer was recently published and combined data from 4 tertiary centers in the United States, Netherlands, Italy, and China.[12] The investigators identified 84 men who underwent lymph node dissection for SCC of the penis between 1978 and 2013 and who were found to have positive pelvic lymph nodes (ie, pN3). In this cohort, 36 men received adjuvant chemotherapy, with a majority (78%) treated with platinum-based regimens (most commonly docetaxel, cisplatin, and 5-fluorouracil [TPF]), whereas 48 were not. At a median follow-up of just over 12 months, median overall survival was significantly greater in those who had received chemotherapy compared with those who had not (21.7 months vs 10.1 months, $P = .048$) (**Fig. 1**). Furthermore, receipt of adjuvant chemotherapy (hazard ratio [HR] = 0.40 [0.19–0.87], $P = .021$) was the sole independent predictor of overall survival in a multivariable analysis adjusting for age, pathologic stage, bilaterality of nodal disease, and timing of pelvic surgery.

There are several important limitations of this study, however, the most important being that men who had received salvage chemotherapy after disease recurrence were excluded, which may have led to a systematic bias. The group who had not received adjuvant chemotherapy likely included men who had been unable to receive it owing to rapid postoperative disease recurrence or poor postoperative recovery. In contrast, the group who did receive adjuvant chemotherapy was probably enriched by men who had recovered quickly after surgery (and were thus able to tolerate chemotherapy) and then never recurred, thereby never requiring salvage chemotherapy. In addition to this and potentially other selection biases, the study was inadequately powered for a multivariable analysis.

Other data on the role of adjuvant chemotherapy for pathologic node-positive penile cancer come from smaller, single-center studies. The earliest data on adjuvant treatment came from a pilot study in Milan, Italy, that was published in the late 1980s.[13] Twelve men who had undergone unilateral or bilateral lymphadenectomy for penile cancer, including 5 who had pelvic nodal disease, received weekly vincristine, bleomycin, and methotrexate (VBM) for 12 weeks, with 11 of the 12 patients (92%) alive and disease-free at a median

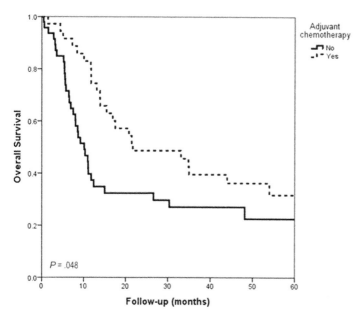

Fig. 1. Overall survival stratified by receipt of adjuvant (adj.) chemotherapy in chemotherapy-naïve men with pelvic node-positive penile cancer. (*From* Sharma P, Djajadiningrat R, Zargar-Shoshtari K, et al. Adjuvant chemotherapy is associated with improved overall survival in pelvic node-positive penile cancer after lymph node dissection: a multi-institutional study. Urol Oncol 2015;33(11):496.e20; with permission.)

Number at risk						
No adj. chemo (n = 48)	26	18	17	16	15	15
Yes adj. chemo (n = 36)	31	21	18	15	14	13

follow-up of 42 months. There were 2 cases of bleomycin-induced lung injury, however.

Poorer survival outcomes were reported in a small German case series evaluating adjuvant bleomycin, methotrexate, and cisplatin (BMP). Three of 8 men (38%) with pN1-3 disease were alive and free of disease at a mean of 4.5 years after adjuvant treatment, and 1 individual died as a result of lung toxicity secondary to bleomycin.[14] Doublet (rather than triplet) chemotherapy has also been investigated in the adjuvant setting in an effort to reduce toxicity and this approach was shown to achieve good outcomes in a retrospective study from Mumbai, India. A combination of paclitaxel with either carboplatin or cisplatin was used in 19 men with high-risk locally advanced disease (defined as perinodal extension, bilateral nodal involvement, and pelvic node disease and those with incomplete surgical resection) and produced a 2-year overall survival of 68%.[15] At a median follow-up of 15 months, 6 men (32%) had suffered a locoregional relapse, and 3 died (2 due to disease and 1 treatment-related death secondary to diarrhea and neutropenic fever).

The latest data on adjuvant therapy from the Milan group recorded disappointingly poor outcomes in 19 men with pN2 or pN3 disease who received adjuvant cisplatin and 5-FU in combination with a taxane (paclitaxel or docetaxel), termed TPF, with a 2-year disease-free survival of 37%.[16] Additionally, there was substantial hematologic toxicity, with 6 cases of grade 3 or 4 anemia, neutropenia, or thrombocytopenia. These investigators recently evaluated factors associated with better outcomes in men who received adjuvant TPF and found that that p53 immunohistochemical positivity in the nodal metastasis seemed to predict for poorer disease-free survival (HR = 3.76 [0.78–17.96], P = .096) and overall survival (HR = 4.29 [0.89–20.57], P = .067) in multivariate analyses, although results did not reach statistical significance.[17] These preliminary results are hypothesis generating and merit further study in ongoing efforts to determine which men with advanced penile cancer might benefit most from adjuvant therapy.

Summary

Table 2 summarizes the current available evidence on the role of adjuvant chemotherapy in node-positive penile cancer. There are no randomized data, and reported follow-up is short, which raises questions on whether a survival benefit from adjuvant chemotherapy can be durable, while attempts to define predictive and prognostic factors are at a very early stage. Although a majority of patients received a platinum-based regimen,

Table 2
Summary of studies on adjuvant chemotherapy in node-positive penile cancer

Citation	Patient Cohort	N	Regimen	Median (Mean) Follow-up, mo	Survival Outcomes	Toxicity
Pizzocaro & Piva,[13] 1988	Involved inguinal and/or pelvic nodes	12	VBM	42	• 11 Alive and disease-free • 1 Died of disease	Bleomycin-induced lung damage (n = 2)
Hakenberg et al,[14] 2006	pTx pN1-3 M0	8	BMP	(54)	• 3 Alive and disease-free • 4 Died of disease • 1 Treatment-related death	• Treatment-related death (n = 1) • Any grade 3 or 4 (n = 24/45)
Noronha et al,[15] 2012	High-risk nodal disease (PNE, bilateral nodal disease, pelvic nodal disease, R1 resection)	19	TP	15	• 2-Year OS = 68% • 6 Locoregional relapses • 2 Died of disease • 1 Treatment-related death	• Treatment-related death (n = 1) • Any grade 3 or 4 (n = 6)
Nicolai et al,[16] 2015	≥pN2 M0	19	• TPF (n = 16) • Paclitaxel-PF (n = 3)	N/A	• 10 Alive and disease-free • 8 Died of disease • 1 Died of other cause • 2-Year DFS of 37%	Any grade 3 or 4 (n = 10)
Sharma et al,[12] 2015	pN3 M0	36	• TPF (n = 18) • PF (n = 8) • VBM (n = 8) • TIP (n = 1) • BMP (n = 1)	12	• mOS = 21.7 mo (vs 10.1 mo in a cohort of 48 men who did not receive adjuvant chemotherapy), P = .048 • Adjuvant chemotherapy HR for OS = 0.40 (0.19–0.87), P = .021	N/A

Abbreviations: DFS, disease-free survival; mOS, median overall survival; N/A, not available; PF, cisplatin, 5-FU; PNE, perinodal extension; OS, overall survival; TP, paclitaxel, cis/carboplatin.

the optimal combination (doublet or triplet) is also yet to be defined. Nevertheless, taken together, adjuvant platinum-based therapy does have a role in the management of chemotherapy-naïve patients with pelvic node-positive penile cancer, given the premise that it offers the possibility of long-term survival in this cohort of men who might otherwise be expected to relapse without adjuvant treatment.

MULTIMODAL APPROACH TO BULKY OR UNRESECTABLE NODAL DISEASE

Surgery alone is rarely a curative option in men with advanced inguinal or pelvic nodal disease. Bilateral, numerous, and bulky inguinal involvement; extranodal extension; and the presence of pelvic nodal metastases are known prognostic factors in penile cancer, and a multimodal approach is desirable in treating patients with these features.[3,18,19]

Neoadjuvant chemotherapy offers the ability to downstage disease and thereby enable surgical resection among responders, even among men with advanced penile cancer. Data from the Southwest Oncology Group phase II trial of BMP included examples of bulky inguinal lymph node disease that had a partial response (4 patients) or complete response (2 patients).[20] Details of postchemotherapy surgery were not reported in that study, and although a response was seen in nearly 1 in 3 men (including lymph node and distant metastases), toxicity with BMP was significant, with 5 treatment-related deaths (from infection or pulmonary complications) among 45 registered patients.

Building on these results, Leijte and colleagues[21] from the Netherlands reported the outcomes in 20 patients who received neoadjuvant chemotherapy for M0 penile cancer between 1972 and 2005. Although there was heterogeneity in the regimens used (VBM; BMP; 5-FU and cisplatin; cisplatin and irinotecan; and single-agent bleomycin), an overall response (either complete or partial response) was seen in 12 of 19 evaluable patients (63%). Importantly, 8 of the 9 responders who went on to undergo lymphadenectomy had durable long-term survival with no evidence of disease recurrence at a median follow-up of 20 months, with 2 having a pathologic complete response (pCR) on postoperative histology. Response to neoadjuvant therapy was also prognostic, with a 56% 5-year overall survival in men who responded, whereas all nonresponders had died within 9 months of treatment.

The similarities between SCC of the penis and head and neck have prompted study of alternative neoadjuvant regimens. The Milan group reported retrospective data on their experience with neoadjuvant TPF, the overall results of which seem slightly poorer compared with the Dutch data. A median of 4 cycles of TPF was administered to 28 men with clinical N3 disease, producing an overall response rate of 43%.[16] Of the 22 men who subsequently underwent surgery, 7 (32%) were alive and disease-free at a median follow-up of more than 12 months, including 2 of the 4 who achieved a pCR. In the entire cohort, however, 12 men relapsed and 9 died of disease, with an additional 3 deaths due to other causes, including 1 treatment-related death from cardiac toxicity. Response to treatment was also not associated with survival, although the study was underpowered to assess this.

These retrospective data served to confirm that neoadjuvant chemotherapy is feasible and potentially effective as part of a multimodal approach against advanced penile cancer. Four prospective studies have added to the evidence base but the small numbers of patients they have accrued make it difficult to generate robust conclusions. The European Organisation for Research and Treatment of Cancer (EORTC) conducted a multicenter phase II study of neoadjuvant irinotecan in combination with cisplatin in 7 men with T3 or N1-2 disease.[22] A median of 4 cycles of treatment was administered, and 2 men (29%) achieved a clinical response, with a pCR seen in 3 men who underwent postchemotherapy resection.

Investigators at the University of Texas MD Anderson Cancer Center conducted the largest prospective study of neoadjuvant chemotherapy for locally advanced disease in the form of a phase II trial enrolling 30 men with clinical stage Tx N2-3 M0 disease, a majority of whom (70%) had clinical N3 disease at baseline.[23] Patients received 4 cycles of paclitaxel, ifosfamide, and cisplatin (TIP) prior to planned bilateral inguinal and unilateral or bilateral pelvic lymphadenectomy. The treatment was well tolerated, with a majority of men completing all 4 planned cycles and grade 3 infection the most commonly observed adverse event (on 5 occasions). All but 4 individuals went on to undergo lymphadenectomy, including 22 of the 23 men who completed all 4 cycles of chemotherapy. The objective response rate, measured by Response Evaluation Criteria in Solid Tumors (RECIST), was 50% (with 3 complete responses and 12 partial responses) and 3 men had a pCR (13.6%). Survival outcomes were comparable to those seen in retrospective studies,[16,21] with 9 men (30%) remaining alive and disease-free at a median follow-up of 34 months, with a reported median overall survival within the entire cohort of 17 months. Response to neoadjuvant TIP also predicted for longer time to disease progression and overall survival (**Fig. 2**). Postoperative complications were comparable to those seen in contemporary lymphadenectomy series,[24] suggesting that neoadjuvant chemotherapy did not increase surgical morbidity.

The same investigators subsequently published a follow-up report by retrospectively reviewing results from an additional 31 men with Tx N1-3 M0 disease who underwent neoadjuvant chemotherapy, predominantly with TIP, to produce an overall cohort of 61 patients.[25] This report included 21 men who had undergone a prior inguinal procedure and were being treated for disease recurrence or persistence. There was an impressive overall response rate of 65% (39 of 61 men), and the vast majority (85%) went on to undergo surgery, with 10 men (19%) achieving a pCR; 50% of the chemotherapy responders were alive and disease-free at a median follow-up of more than 5 years, as were 7 of the 10 whose surgery had revealed a pCR, suggesting that this multimodal approach to advanced penile cancer had contributed to the observed long-term survival.

Prospective studies of other platinum-based regimens in the treatment of metastatic penile cancer have not been as successful as the MD Anderson experience with TIP. A well-designed phase II trial in the United Kingdom involving 21 men with

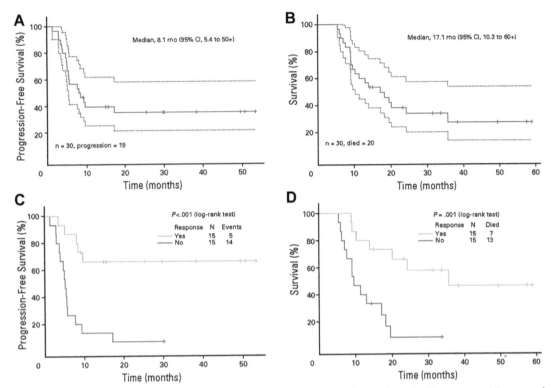

Fig. 2. Kaplan-Meier curves showing (*A*) time to disease progression, (*B*) overall survival in men receiving neoadjuvant TIP, and (*C*) time to progression, and (*D*) overall survival stratified by response to neoadjuvant chemotherapy, respectively. The 95% CIs are shown (*A, B*) with dashed lines above and below. (*From* Pagliaro LC, Williams DL, Daliani D, et al. Neoadjuvant paclitaxel, ifosfamide, and cisplatin chemotherapy for metastatic penile cancer: a phase II study. J Clin Oncol 2010;28(24):3854; with permission.)

Tx N1-3 M0 penile cancer (a majority of whom had N3 disease) aimed to assess response clinically and via RECIST after a planned 3 cycles of TPF and determine how many patients subsequently became operable.[26] The overall response rate was 37% in men with evaluable locally advanced disease, and 5 of 20 patients who were deemed inoperable at trial entry were sufficiently downstaged to proceed with surgery. Toxicity with TPF was substantially greater than that with TIP, however, with more than 2 in 3 patients suffering any grade 3 or 4 adverse events.

The most recent prospective study examining the role of neoadjuvant chemotherapy comes from the Netherlands Cancer Institute and was published in 2015.[27] They used neoadjuvant TPF as part of a nonrandomized institutional study (with a higher dose of cisplatin than that used in the previously described UK TPF phase II trial[26]) in 26 men with T4 and/or N3 disease and aimed at downstaging men sufficiently to permit surgery. Almost half of the cohort completed all of the planned 4 cycles, and complete and partial responses (per RECIST) were seen in 2 and 9 patients, respectively, giving an overall response

rate of 44% in the 25 evaluable patients. An additional 4 men achieved stable disease, and of the 15 individuals in whom stable disease or better was attained, 14 underwent surgery, with 1 patient having a pCR. Taking into consideration the heterogeneity of the cohort (almost half were treated for recurrent disease, thereby potentially selecting for more aggressive disease biology), survival outcomes were still disappointing. Only 4 men (15%) were alive and disease-free at a median follow-up of 30 months and median overall survival was 10 months, compared with the 17 months seen with TIP. Furthermore, 6 men discontinued therapy owing to toxicity, and all enrolled men experienced at least grade 2 or higher toxicity.

Summary

Table 3 summarizes currently published evidence on the use of neoadjuvant chemotherapy for locally advanced penile cancer. A response rate of 29% to 65% has been seen with the use of neoadjuvant chemotherapy and it is an important part of the multimodal approach to treat advanced penile cancer. The disease seems most sensitive

Table 3
Summary of studies on neoadjuvant chemotherapy for unresectable nodal disease

Citation	Patient Cohort	N	Regimen(s)	Median Follow-up, mo	Response Rate, %	Underwent Surgery (%)	Pathologic Complete Response at Surgery (% of Those Operated)	Survival Outcomes
Leijte et al,[21] 2007	Tx N0-3 M0	20	BMP (n = 10) VBM (n = 5) Bleomycin (n = 3) PF (n = 1) Cisplatin-irinotecan (n = 1)	23	63	9 (45)	2 (22)	• 5-Y OS = 32% • 8 of 9 undergoing surgery alive and disease-free at median follow-up of 20 mo
Theodore et al,[22] 2008	T3 N1-2 M0	7	Cisplatin-irinotecan	N/A	29	3 (43)	3 (100)	N/A
Pagliaro et al,[23] 2010	Tx N2-3 M0	30	TIP	34	50	22 (73)	3 (14)	• 9 Alive and disease-free • mOS = 17 mo
Dickstein et al,[25] 2016[a]	Tx N1-3 M0 (including prior inguinal procedure)	61	TIP (n = 53) TP, PF, BMP (n = 7)	N/A	65	52 (85)	10 (19)	• 20 Alive and disease-free at 5 y • 32 Died of disease at 5 y
Nicolai et al,[16] 2015	Tx N3 M0 (including 5 with relapsed disease)	28	TPF (n = 23) Paclitaxel-PF (n = 5)	N/A	43	22 (79)	4 (18)	• 8 Alive and disease-free • 9 Died of disease • 2-Year DFS = 7%
Djajadiningrat et al,[27] 2015	T4 and/or N3 (including 12 with relapsed disease)	26	TPF	30	44	14 (54)	N/A	• 4 Alive and disease-free • 13 Died of disease • mOS = 10 mo • 1-Year OS = 46% • 2-Year OS = 27%

Abbreviations: DFS, disease-free survival; mOS, median overall survival; N/A, not available; PF, cisplatin, 5-FU; OS, overall survival; TIP, paclitaxel ifosfamide, cisplatin; TP, paclitaxel, cisplatin; TP, paclitaxel, cisplatin; TP, paclitaxel, cis/carboplatin.

[a] This study included patients from Pagliaro and colleagues, 2010.[23]

Data from Pagliaro LC, Williams DL, Daliani D, et al. Neoadjuvant paclitaxel, ifosfamide, and cisplatin chemotherapy for metastatic penile cancer: a phase II study. J Clin Oncol 2010;28(24):3851–7.

to platinum-based therapy, with TIP offering the highest response rates. Translating response into a durable survival benefit, however, has proved difficult and optimizing this multimodal approach to do so requires further study. Nevertheless, current European Association of Urology[28] and National Comprehensive Cancer Network[29] guidelines recommend the use, wherever feasible, of a triplet regimen, including cisplatin and a taxane, followed by consolidation surgery in men with bulky or initially unresectable nodal disease who respond to neoadjuvant chemotherapy.

IS THERE A ROLE FOR CHEMORADIOTHERAPY?

The question of whether chemoradiotherapy may be a feasible option for men with locally advanced and regionally metastatic penile cancer has been raised owing to the superiority of this approach compared with single-modality therapy alone in the treatment of locally advanced SCCs of the vulva and anus, 2 rare perineal tumors that share anatomic and biologic characteristics with penile cancer.[5,6,30] Concurrent chemoradiation has also gained traction because neoadjuvant radiotherapy has been shown to reduce inguinal recurrence rates in men with bulky nodal disease,[31] offering the possibility of synergistic activity with neoadjuvant chemotherapy.

The data on chemoradiotherapy for advanced penile cancer are limited to case reports and case series. The sole multicenter study examining chemoradiation collated data between 2000 and 2012 from 5 tertiary centers in the United States, Canada, and Italy.[32] In this 26-patient cohort, including 16 men with clinical stage IV disease and 5 with M1 disease, a majority received cisplatin-based chemotherapy together with a median dose of 4900 cGy to involved disease areas. Accepting that most patients had stage IV disease at outset and that men with relapsed disease were also included, however, clinical outcomes were disappointing: 1-year overall survival was 37% in men with M0 disease, a figure that is less than that achieved with neoadjuvant chemotherapy alone followed by surgical consolidation.[23]

The extreme paucity of data on chemoradiation for advanced penile cancer, therefore, means that this approach is currently investigational, requiring further evaluation within clinical trials, a sentiment that is reflected in consensus guidelines.[28] It is, however, a reasonable treatment option for patients who refuse surgery or are deemed inoperable despite receiving neoadjuvant systemic chemotherapy.

THE NEED FOR MULTICENTER COLLABORATION

The rarity of penile cancer means that international and multicenter collaboration is an absolute necessity to enable sufficient accrual of patients into clinical trials such that clinically meaningful results may be produced. The 4 phase II trials of neoadjuvant chemotherapy[22,23,26,27] accrued a combined total of 84 patients across 15 years. The UK study[26] was able to recruit 21 men in just 15 months, which was in part due to the enrollment of patients treated at 9 specialist centers, highlighting the role that collaboration between centers of expertise can play in improving patient recruitment into trials for a rare cancer.

To this end, the UK National Institute for Health Research Cancer Research Network, Cancer Research UK, the US National Cancer Institute, and the EORTC came together in 2011 to form the International Rare Cancers Initiative (IRCI), which aims to facilitate the development of international clinical trials for patients with rare cancers, including penile cancer.[33] The International Penile Advanced Cancer Trial (InPACT; NCT02305654) (Fig. 3)[34] is the first such IRCI trial for penile cancer and plans to recruit 400 men with locally advanced (ie, nodally metastatic) penile cancer. Men first will be randomized either to standard surgery (inguinal lymphadenectomy), neoadjuvant chemotherapy (with TIP) followed by consolidation surgery, or neoadjuvant chemoradiotherapy (45 Gy in 25 fractions over 5 weeks with weekly cisplatin as a radiosensitizer) followed by surgery. Those who are deemed at high risk of recurrence after inguinal lymphadenectomy will subsequently be randomized to receive either prophylactic pelvic lymphadenectomy or no further surgery. The primary outcome will be overall survival, with secondary outcomes measures, including disease-specific survival, pathologic complete remission rates, quality of life, and surgical complication rates. This trial, which is yet to open, represents a landmark event in the penile cancer field and will provide the first randomized data in the advanced disease setting. It is also hoped that it will open the door to further multiinstitutional collaboration, which is crucial in providing physicians with a robust evidence base on which to base treatment decisions for men with advanced penile cancer.

SUMMARY

Although penile cancer remains a rare disease, significant progress has been made in developing an evidence base to support the use of a

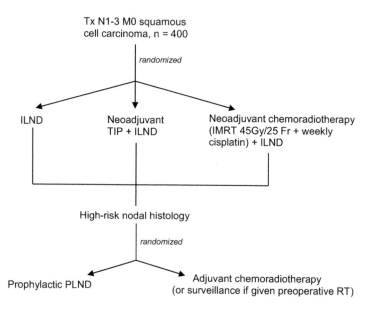

Tx N1-3 M0 squamous cell carcinoma, n = 400

randomized

ILND

Neoadjuvant TIP + ILND

Neoadjuvant chemoradiotherapy (IMRT 45Gy/25 Fr + weekly cisplatin) + ILND

High-risk nodal histology

randomized

Prophylactic PLND

Adjuvant chemoradiotherapy (or surveillance if given preoperative RT)

Fig. 3. InPACT trial design. ILND, inguinal lymph node dissection; IMRT, intensity-modulated radiotherapy; PLND, pelvic lymph node dissection; RT, radiotherapy.

multimodal approach to regionally metastatic disease (**Fig. 4**). Prospective data have shown that neoadjuvant chemotherapy, with TIP seeming the most active regimen followed by surgical consolidation, has the potential to lead to a durable long-term survival, at least in some men. Adjuvant chemotherapy also improves outcomes for men who have undergone lymphadenectomy for resectable disease and who are chemotherapy naïve.

There remain several unanswered questions in the treatment of advanced penile cancer. What factors predict for response to (neo)adjuvant chemotherapy and are prognostic for survival? Is there a role for concurrent chemoradiotherapy? Is it possible to stratify patients by their molecular status or HPV positivity, and how can newer targeted therapies be integrated into the current multimodal treatment paradigm? The answers to these questions will come from international

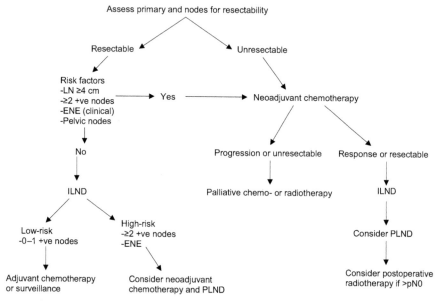

Assess primary and nodes for resectability

Resectable

Unresectable

Risk factors
-LN ≥4 cm
-≥2 +ve nodes
-ENE (clinical)
-Pelvic nodes

Yes

Neoadjuvant chemotherapy

No

Progression or unresectable

Response or resectable

ILND

Palliative chemo- or radiotherapy

ILND

Low-risk
-0–1 +ve nodes

High-risk
-≥2 +ve nodes
-ENE

Consider PLND

Adjuvant chemotherapy or surveillance

Consider neoadjuvant chemotherapy and PLND

Consider postoperative radiotherapy if >pN0

Fig. 4. Summary of current approach to multimodal therapy in men with locoregionally advanced squamous cell penile cancer. +ve, positive; ENE, extranodal extension; ILND, inguinal lymph node dissection; LN, lymph node(s); PLND, pelvic lymph node dissection.

collaboration across clinical trials, of which the authors hope InPACT to be the first of many.

REFERENCES

1. Siegel RL, Miller KD, Jemal A. Cancer statistics, 2016. CA Cancer J Clin 2016;66(1):7–30.
2. Goodman MT, Hernandez BY, Shvetsov YB. Demographic and pathologic differences in the incidence of invasive penile cancer in the United States, 1995-2003. Cancer Epidemiol Biomarkers Prev 2007; 16(9):1833–9.
3. Ravi R. Correlation between the extent of nodal involvement and survival following groin dissection for carcinoma of the penis. Br J Urol 1993; 72(5 Pt 2):817–9.
4. Bernier J, Domenge C, Ozsahin M, et al. Postoperative irradiation with or without concomitant chemotherapy for locally advanced head and neck cancer. N Engl J Med 2004;350(19):1945–52.
5. Ajani JA, Winter KA, Gunderson LL, et al. Fluorouracil, mitomycin, and radiotherapy vs fluorouracil, cisplatin, and radiotherapy for carcinoma of the anal canal: a randomized controlled trial. JAMA 2008;299(16):1914–21.
6. Montana GS, Thomas GM, Moore DH, et al. Preoperative chemo-radiation for carcinoma of the vulva with N2/N3 nodes: a gynecologic oncology group study. Int J Radiat Oncol Biol Phys 2000; 48(4):1007–13.
7. Hakenberg OW, Wirth MP. Issues in the treatment of penile carcinoma. A short review. Urol Int 1999; 62(4):229–33.
8. Pizzocaro G, Piva L, Bandieramonte G, et al. Up-to-date management of carcinoma of the penis. Eur Urol 1997;32(1):5–15.
9. Leijte JA, Kirrander P, Antonini N, et al. Recurrence patterns of squamous cell carcinoma of the penis: recommendations for follow-up based on a two-centre analysis of 700 patients. Eur Urol 2008; 54(1):161–8.
10. Ficarra V, Akduman B, Bouchot O, et al. Prognostic factors in penile cancer. Urology 2010; 76(2 Suppl 1):S66–73.
11. Slaton JW, Morgenstern N, Levy DA, et al. Tumor stage, vascular invasion and the percentage of poorly differentiated cancer: independent prognosticators for inguinal lymph node metastasis in penile squamous cancer. J Urol 2001;165(4):1138–42.
12. Sharma P, Djajadiningrat R, Zargar-Shoshtari K, et al. Adjuvant chemotherapy is associated with improved overall survival in pelvic node-positive penile cancer after lymph node dissection: a multi-institutional study. Urol Oncol 2015;33(11): 496.e17-23.
13. Pizzocaro G, Piva L. Adjuvant and neoadjuvant vincristine, bleomycin, and methotrexate for inguinal metastases from squamous cell carcinoma of the penis. Acta Oncol 1988;27(6b):823–4.
14. Hakenberg OW, Nippgen JB, Froehner M, et al. Cisplatin, methotrexate and bleomycin for treating advanced penile carcinoma. BJU Int 2006;98(6): 1225–7.
15. Noronha V, Patil V, Ostwal V, et al. Role of paclitaxel and platinum-based adjuvant chemotherapy in high-risk penile cancer. Urol Ann 2012;4(3):150–3.
16. Nicolai N, Sangalli LM, Necchi A, et al. A combination of Cisplatin and 5-Fluorouracil with a taxane in patients who underwent lymph node dissection for nodal metastases from squamous cell carcinoma of the penis: treatment outcome and survival analyses in neoadjuvant and adjuvant settings. Clin Genitourin Cancer 2015. [Epub ahead of print].
17. Necchi A, Lo Vullo S, Nicolai N, et al. Prognostic factors of adjuvant chemotherapy with taxane, cisplatin, and 5FU combination (TPF) in patients (pts) with nodal metastases of penile squamous cell carcinoma (PSCC). J Clin Oncol 2016;34(Suppl 2S) [abstract: 479].
18. Pandey D, Mahajan V, Kannan RR. Prognostic factors in node-positive carcinoma of the penis. J Surg Oncol 2006;93(2):133–8.
19. Novara G, Galfano A, De Marco V, et al. Prognostic factors in squamous cell carcinoma of the penis. Nat Clin Pract Urol 2007;4(3):140–6.
20. Haas GP, Blumenstein BA, Gagliano RG, et al. Cisplatin, methotrexate and bleomycin for the treatment of carcinoma of the penis: a Southwest Oncology Group study. J Urol 1999;161(6):1823–5.
21. Leijte JA, Kerst JM, Bais E, et al. Neoadjuvant chemotherapy in advanced penile carcinoma. Eur Urol 2007;52(2):488–94.
22. Theodore C, Skoneczna I, Bodrogi I, et al. A phase II multicentre study of irinotecan (CPT 11) in combination with cisplatin (CDDP) in metastatic or locally advanced penile carcinoma (EORTC PROTOCOL 30992). Ann Oncol 2008;19(7):1304–7.
23. Pagliaro LC, Williams DL, Daliani D, et al. Neoadjuvant paclitaxel, ifosfamide, and cisplatin chemotherapy for metastatic penile cancer: a phase II study. J Clin Oncol 2010;28(24):3851–7.
24. Bevan-Thomas R, Slaton JW, Pettaway CA. Contemporary morbidity from lymphadenectomy for penile squamous cell carcinoma: the M.D. Anderson Cancer Center Experience. J Urol 2002; 167(4):1638–42.
25. Dickstein RJ, Munsell MF, Pagliaro LC, et al. Prognostic factors influencing survival from regionally advanced squamous cell carcinoma of the penis after preoperative chemotherapy. BJU Int 2016;117(1):118–25.
26. Nicholson S, Hall E, Harland SJ, et al. Phase II trial of docetaxel, cisplatin and 5FU chemotherapy in locally advanced and metastatic penis cancer (CRUK/09/001). Br J Cancer 2013;109(10):2554–9.

27. Djajadiningrat RS, Bergman AM, van Werkhoven E, et al. Neoadjuvant taxane-based combination chemotherapy in patients with advanced penile cancer. Clin Genitourin Cancer 2015;13(1):44–9.

28. Hakenberg OW, Comperat EM, Minhas S, et al. EAU guidelines on penile cancer: 2014 update. Eur Urol 2015;67(1):142–50.

29. Clark PE, Spiess PE, Agarwal N, et al. Penile cancer: clinical practice guidelines in oncology. J Natl Compr Canc Netw 2013;11(5):594–615.

30. Longpre MJ, Lange PH, Kwon JS, et al. Penile carcinoma: lessons learned from vulvar carcinoma. J Urol 2013;189(1):17–24.

31. Ravi R, Chaturvedi HK, Sastry DV. Role of radiation therapy in the treatment of carcinoma of the penis. Br J Urol 1994;74(5):646–51.

32. Pond GR, Milowsky MI, Kolinsky MP, et al. Concurrent chemoradiotherapy for men with locally advanced penile squamous cell carcinoma. Clin Genitourin Cancer 2014;12(6):440–6.

33. Keat N, Law K, Seymour M, et al. International rare cancers initiative. Lancet Oncol 2013;14(2):109–10.

34. Nicholson S, Kayes O, Minhas S. Clinical trial strategy for penis cancer. BJU Int 2014;113(6): 852–3.

Emerging Systemic Therapies for the Management of Penile Cancer

Shilpa Gupta, MD[a], Guru Sonpavde, MD[b],*

KEYWORDS

- Penile squamous cell carcinoma • Combined modality therapy • Chemotherapy • Targeted therapy
- EGFR • PD-1 • VEGF

KEY POINTS

- Penile squamous cell carcinoma (PSCC) is a rare cancer in men in developed countries and more common in developing countries.
- Prognosis of metastatic PSCC is dismal, and responses to chemotherapy are short-lived.
- There is an urgent need to incorporate novel targeted and immunotherapy agents in the treatment paradigm.

INTRODUCTION

Penile squamous cell carcinoma (PSCC) is a rare cancer in men in developed countries, with an estimated 2030 new cases of PSCC and 340 deaths in the United States in 2016.[1] The incidence of PSCC is higher in the developing countries of Asia, Africa, and South America.[2] The most common age of presentation is between 50 and 70 years.[3]

PSCC is an aggressive disease, spreading locally through lymphatic channels and subsequently to distant sites. The survival outcomes of patients with penile cancer depend on the presence or absence of lymph node involvement.[4,5] The 5-year survival rate is more than 85% for patients with negative lymph nodes and 29% to 40% with positive nodes and 0% for those with pelvic lymph node involvement.[5] Although surgical excision is the standard of care for patients with palpable inguinal lymph nodes less than 4 cm in size, for those with inguinal lymph nodes greater than 4 cm, fixed nodes, or involvement of pelvic lymph nodes, multimodality treatment with systemic chemotherapy, surgery, and radiation is generally offered.[6] Notably, multiple therapeutic conundrums exist because of the absence of randomized trials. The International Rare Tumors Initiative has launched the International Penile Advanced Cancer Trial (InPACT) trial for patients with inguinal lymph node metastases to elucidate the role of neoadjuvant therapy using chemotherapy or chemoradiotherapy compared with no neoadjuvant therapy. Additionally, the role of pelvic lymph node dissection following surgery and inguinal lymph node dissection will be investigated (NCT02305654).[7]

Successful treatment of advanced PSCC with regional and systemic metastases remains a challenge; given the lack of randomized trials in PSCC,

Disclosures: Advisory board of Genentech, speakers bureau for Genentech (S. Gupta), research support to institution from Onyx, Bayer, Celgene, Pfizer, Merck, Boehringer-Ingelheim; advisory board of Merck, Genentech, Sanofi, Pfizer, Novartis, Argos, Agensys, Bayer; honorarium from Uptodate for author fees and from clinical care options for speaker fees; travel costs covered by Elsevier and Dava Oncology (G. Sonpavde).

[a] Department of Hematology, Oncology and Transplantation, University of Minnesota, Minneapolis, MN 55455, USA; [b] Section of Medical Oncology, Department of Medicine, UAB Comprehensive Cancer Center, 1802 6th Avenue South, NP2540B, Birmingham, AL 35294, USA
* Corresponding author.
E-mail address: gsonpavde@uabmc.edu

Urol Clin N Am 43 (2016) 481–491
http://dx.doi.org/10.1016/j.ucl.2016.06.009
0094-0143/16/© 2016 Elsevier Inc. All rights reserved.

current therapy options are based on small prospective trials and retrospective studies.[8,9] Cisplatin-containing multi-agent systemic chemotherapy regimens are commonly used as first-line treatment of patients with advanced/metastatic PSCC. There are no standard second-line treatment options, and only marginal responses are observed with single-agent paclitaxel.[10] Novel treatment approaches with targeted therapies and immunotherapies are urgently required to improve the outcomes in PSCC refractory to standard therapy. This review highlights the current standard therapies and the role for novel therapies that warrant further studies.

SYSTEMIC CHEMOTHERAPY
Chemotherapy for Advanced/Metastatic Penile Squamous Cell Carcinoma

First-line chemotherapy
Monotherapy with cisplatin, bleomycin, and methotrexate in PSCC was attempted in the early 1970s; but response rates were modest between 0% and 27% (**Table 1**).[11–13] Cisplatin displayed a 15.4% response rate with a median survival of 4.7 months.[11] Bleomycin had modest activity as well and caused major side effects, including pulmonary toxicity.[12,14] One case of complete response was seen with high-dose methotrexate.[15]

Combination chemotherapy regimens with 2 or 3 chemotherapeutic agents was attempted to improve outcomes. There were small studies and case reports of patients treated with cisplatin-based combination chemotherapy. Shammas and colleagues[16] showed a partial response in

2 out of 8 patients treated with cisplatin and 5-fluorouracil. The efficacy of cisplatin-5-fluorouracil was evaluated more recently in a larger retrospective study in patients with metastatic PSCC (see **Table 1**).[17] Among the 25 patients with metastatic PSCC treated with cisplatin plus 5-fluorouracil, partial responses and stable responses were observed in 8 (32%) and 10 (40%) patients, respectively, with a disease control rate of 72%. The median progression-free survival (PFS) was 20 weeks, and the median overall survival (OS) was 8 months. The incidence of grade 3 to 4 neutropenia was 20%.[17]

Kattan and colleagues[18] reported one complete response after treatment with combined cisplatin and methotrexate in 3 patients with metastatic PSCC. In a phase 2 European Organization for Research and Treatment of Cancer study by Theodore and colleagues,[19] 28 patients with advanced/metastatic PSCC were treated with the combination of cisplatin and irinotecan (**Table 2**). Patients were treated either in the neoadjuvant setting for T3 or N1-N2 disease with up to 4 cycles or up to 8 cycles for T4 or N3 or M1 disease. Twenty-six eligible patients were evaluated for response; there were 8 responses (30.8%; 2 complete responses and 6 partial responses).[19] The combination of paclitaxel and carboplatin (PCa) demonstrated significant remission in an anecdote of a single patient and the regimen was well tolerated.[20] In a phase II trial, patients with unresected locoregional lymph nodes and/or distant metastases were administered gemcitabine and cisplatin every 2 weeks.[21] The median time to progression (TTP) was 5.48 months, and

Table 1
Key reported studies of chemotherapy for advanced/metastatic penile squamous cell carcinoma

Author	Regimen	Line of Therapy	N	Response
Shammas et al,[16] 1992	Cisplatin, 5-FU	First	8	PR 3 patients
Di Lorenzo et al,[17] 2012	Cisplatin, 5-FU	First	25	PR 8 patients, SD 10 patients
Gagliano et al,[11] 1989	Cisplatin	First	26	PR 4 patients
Dexeus et al,[23] 1991	Bleomycin, methotrexate, cisplatin	First	14	PR 10 patients
Haas et al,[24] 1999	Bleomycin, methotrexate, cisplatin	First	40	CR 5 patients, PR 8 patients
Theodore et al,[19] 2008	Cisplatin, irinotecan	First	26	CR 2 patients, PR 6 patients
Nicholson et al,[28] 2013	Docetaxel, cisplatin, 5-FU	First	26	CR 2 patients, PR 8 patients
Pizzocaro et al,[81] 2009	Paclitaxel, cisplatin, 5-FU	First	3	PR 2 patients
Di Lorenzo et al,[10] 2011	Paclitaxel	Second	25	PR 5 patients

Abbreviations: CR, complete response; 5-FU, 5-fluorouracil; PR, partial response; SD, stable disease.

Table 2
Key reported studies of neoadjuvant chemotherapy for penile squamous cell carcinoma

Author	Regimen	N	Response
Pizzocaro & Piva,[32] 1988	BVM	5	PR 3 patients
Leijte et al,[27] 2007	BMP, BVM, CF, CI	20	PR 12 patients
Bermejo et al,[31] 2007	ITP, BMP, PCa	10	CR 4 patients, PR 1 patient, SD 5 patients, pathologic CR 3 patients
Pagliaro et al,[33] 2010	ITP	30	Clinical CR 3 patients, PR 12 patients, SD 9 patients; pathologic CR 3 patients

Abbreviations: BMP, bleomycin, methotrexate, cisplatin; BVM, bleomycin, vincristine, methotrexate; CF, cisplatin, 5-fluorouracil; CR, complete response; ITP, ifosfamide, paclitaxel, cisplatin; PCa, paclitaxel, carboplatin; PR, partial response; RR, response rate; SD, stable disease.

the median OS was 14.98 months. However, the trial did not meet the target of 5 responses in the first phase of 25 patients (because a response rate of 20% was considered poorly effective); the regimen was not recommended for further development. There is other anecdotal evidence for the activity of cisplatin and gemcitabine in 2 patients with metastatic PSCC.[22]

In 1991 Dexeus and colleagues[23] reported the activity of a triplet combination of bleomycin, methotrexate, and cisplatin (BMP) in advanced/metastatic in patients with PSCC and demonstrated a response in 10 of 14 patients (72%), with moderate side effects (see **Table 2**). However, the toxicities seemed prohibitive in subsequent studies with the BMP regimen. In a large prospective Southwest Oncology Group multicenter study involving 45 patients with advanced/metastatic PSCC, Haas and colleagues[24] reported their experience with the BMP regimen (see **Table 2**). Out of the 40 patients evaluable for response, there were 5 complete and 8 partial responses (32.5% overall response rate). Unfortunately, there were 5 treatment-related deaths in this study (13.9%); the 6 other patients had at least one life-threatening toxic episode.[24] Hakenberg and colleagues[25] had reported their experience in 5 patients with metastatic PSCC

who received BMP; this regimen showed minimal response, with all 5 patients dying within 5 months of treatment. Similar findings of moderate efficacy and high toxicity were reported in other studies evaluating BMP.[26,27] Based on these findings, the BMP regimen is no longer recommended.

Triplet chemotherapy regimens without bleomycin have demonstrated better therapeutic indices. The efficacy of a triplet regimen consisting of docetaxel, cisplatin-5-fluorouracil (TPF) was studied in advanced PSCC.[28] Ten of 26 evaluable patients (38.5%) responded, and the regimen did not attain the predetermined threshold to trigger further research; but 2 patients with locally advanced disease exhibited complete remission. However, 65.5% of patients experienced grade 3/4 adverse events, which led the investigators to abandon further development of this regimen and not support the routine use of TPF. Nevertheless, owing to the complete responses seen, TPF may be appropriate in the neoadjuvant setting before planned radical surgery with curative intent.

In a retrospective study of 140 men with advanced PSCC receiving first-line systemic therapy for unresectable or metastatic disease, visceral metastases and Eastern Cooperative Oncology Group-Performance Status (ECOG-PS) of 1 or greater were poor prognostic factors.[29] Interestingly, patients receiving cisplatin-based regimens exhibited better outcomes compared with non–cisplatin-based regimens even after adjusting for prognostic factors. These data suggest that a cisplatin-based regimen should be preferred, although the contrary view may be to administer tolerable regimens because none of the regimens seem potentially curative except in the perioperative state.

Salvage chemotherapy

There is no established second-line therapy for metastatic PSCC, and taxanes have been used with moderate activity.[10] Di Lorenzo and colleagues[10] performed a phase 2 study using 3-weekly paclitaxel at a dose of 175 mg/m^2 in 25 patients with pretreated metastatic PSCC. Partial responses were observed in 5 out of 25 patients (20%); the median PFS was 11 weeks; the median OS was 23 weeks. This study demonstrated that paclitaxel was moderately active in relapsed patients and was reasonably well tolerated.[10]

Vinflunine, a third-generation synthetic vinca alkaloid chemotherapeutic agent with antiangiogenic properties, is currently approved as salvage therapy for metastatic urothelial carcinoma in multiple countries (but not in the United States).[30] A Phase II Trial of Vinflunine Chemotherapy in Locally-advanced and Metastatic Carcinoma of the Penis (VINCaP) is ongoing in locally advanced/metastatic PSCC, and results will probably be available in 2018 (NCT02057913) (see **Table 4**).

Neoadjuvant Chemotherapy

Small retrospective and prospective studies evaluated bleomycin-containing regimens, including bleomycin-vincristine-methotrexate (BVM) and BMP, in neoadjuvant fashion for those with bulky regional disease with adenopathy stage N2-N3 (see **Table 2**).[27,31,32] Pizzocaro and Piva[32] used a weekly BVM regimen in a neoadjuvant fashion in 5 patients with fixed inguinal nodes. Patients were treated with 12 weekly courses. Partial responses were seen in 3 of 5 patients; but 2 patients developed pulmonary fibrosis form bleomycin, leading to treatment discontinuation.[32] In the study by Lejite and colleagues,[27] one treatment-related death was reported. In the retrospective study by Bermejo and colleagues,[31] neoadjuvant use of PCa in 2 patients showed favorable outcomes with long-term survival in patients undergoing lymph node dissection after chemotherapy. In the study by Bermejo and colleagues,[31] the neoadjuvant ifosfamide, paclitaxel, and cisplatin (ITP) regimen was also used with favorable outcomes after surgery (see **Table 2**).

Thereafter, Pagliaro and colleagues[33] evaluated ITP in a phase 2 trial recruiting 30 patients with locally advanced PSCC with bulky lymphadenopathy with clinical stage N2-3 (see **Table 2**). Neoadjuvant treatment with 4 cycles of ITP was planned every 3 to 4 weeks. Twenty-three patients (76.7%) completed the planned 4 courses of chemotherapy; 15 out of 30 patients (50.0%) had an objective response, and 22 (73.3%) subsequently underwent surgery. Three patients (10%) had a complete pathologic response. Nine patients (30.0%) remained alive and disease free after a median follow-up of 34 months. The median TTP was 8.1 months, and the median OS was 17.1 months.[33] Patients with bilateral residual tumor at resection or extracapsular extension into extranodal tissue or involvement of resected skin or subcutaneous tissue had a worse TTP and OS compared with those who did not. Also, there was a significant improvement in TTP and OS seen in patients who had an objective response to chemotherapy compared with those who did not.[33] In an updated report of 54 patients who received ITP, 39 patients (65%) exhibited a partial response or greater and long-term survival was associated with pathologic response.[34] Given the efficacy of ITP in the neoadjuvant setting, this regimen may be considered acceptable even in the metastatic/unresectable context.

Adjuvant Chemotherapy

There are limited data on the use of adjuvant chemotherapy in PSCC. In the only prospective study done so far, Pizzocaro and Piva[32] evaluated the role of adjuvant BVM in PSCC after surgical resection of local disease and inguinal lymph node metastases (**Table 3**). Twelve patients with radically resected inguinal lymph node metastases from PSCC were treated with 12 weekly courses of BVM; only 1 of the 12 patients relapsed after a median follow-up of 42 months, and the 5-year survival rate was 82% with adjuvant chemotherapy compared with 37% in the historic control group.[32]

Pizzocaro and colleagues[35] also showed that use of 3 cycles of adjuvant cisplatin and 5-fluorouracil in patients with pN2-3 disease improved outcomes. In another retrospective review, adjuvant treatment with paclitaxel and cisplatin also improved outcomes.[36] Hakenberg and colleagues[25] retrospectively evaluated the use of BMP in 13 patients with PSCC, of whom 8 had undergone resection of local and nodal disease. Three out of 8 patients had no evidence of disease after a mean range of 54 months, whereas 4 died of disease progression after a mean of 11 months, and one died of treatment-related toxicity. Although this study showed that patients with minimal disease after surgery may benefit from adjuvant BMV, the toxicity was very high, including risk of death.[25]

Use of the adjuvant ITP regimen in PSCC was retrospectively evaluated at a single center in Ireland and reported in abstract form.[37] Three

Table 3 Key reported studies of adjuvant chemotherapy for penile squamous cell carcinoma			
Author	**Regimen**	**N**	**Response**
Pizzocaro & Piva[32] 1988	BVM	12	11 patients remained disease free at median follow-up of 42 mo
Pizzocaro et al,[35] 1997	BVM or CF	25	84% DFS
Hakenberg et al,[25] 2006	BMP	8	3 patients were disease free at mean 54 mo

Abbreviations: BMP, bleomycin-methotrexate-cisplatin; BVM, bleomycin-vincristine-methotrexate; CF, cisplatin, 5-fluorouracil; DFS, disease-free survival.

patients received adjuvant ITP for 4 cycles; 2 out of these 3 patients received chemotherapy in the adjuvant setting, of which 3 received 4 cycles of ITP regimen. One patient remains disease free at 28 months; one is disease free at 50 months, and 1 is disease free at 6 months.

Given the lack of robust data from prospective trials, the use of adjuvant chemotherapy should be considered in selected patients. The guidelines from the European Association of Urology and the European Society of Medical Oncology recommend use of adjuvant chemotherapy for pN2 or greater disease, and the National Comprehensive Cancer Network's (NCCN) guidelines recommend adjuvant chemotherapy for lymph nodes 4 cm or greater if chemotherapy was not already administered before surgery.[6,38–40]

RECENT INSIGHTS REGARDING TUMOR BIOLOGY FROM GENOMIC STUDIES OF PENILE SQUAMOUS CELL CARCINOMA

Overall, PSCC seems to demonstrate substantial molecular heterogeneity and absence of addiction to a dominant molecular driver (**Fig. 1**). The association of PSCC with human papilloma virus (HPV) 16 and 18, cigarette smoking, and absence of circumcision has been described in the past.[41–46] The Catalogue of Somatic Mutations in Cancer dataset revealed p53 and PIK3CA mutations in 38% and 29% of tumors, respectively.[47] Interestingly, HPV infection seemed to disrupt retinoblastoma protein (RB) and upregulate p16 and p21 but did not correlate with p53 in one study of 148 tumors.[48] Recent studies have reported somatic gene alterations in PSCC. Three studies of modest sample size (tumors from 11–43 patients) reported gene alterations in EGFR, PIK3CA, NOTCH1, CDKN2A, CCND1, AR, JAK2, JAK3, ALK, PTEN, and BRCA2.[49–51] Other modest-sized studies have conducted proteomic and transcriptomics investigations of tumor tissue and provided insights regarding the potential importance of KIT, GNRH, NF-kB, and ERBB2/ERBB3 signaling.[52,53] Collectively, these reports suggest the potential biological importance of the EGFR/HER family, the PI3K pathway, JAK-STAT signaling, and deficits in DNA damage repair due to BRCA alterations in driving PSCC growth and drug resistance. Therefore, inhibitors of these pathways may yield clinical benefits. Unfortunately, the absence of preclinical systems is a

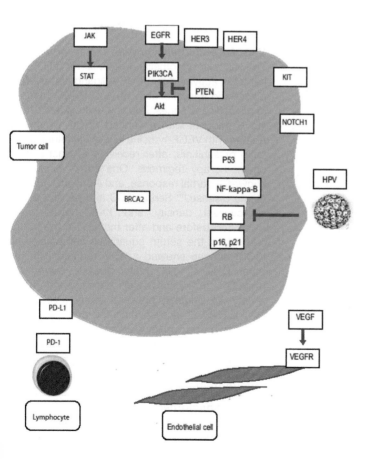

Fig. 1. Potential therapeutic targets in PSCC. Tumor tissue studies indicate the potential role of the EGFR/Her3/Her4, JAK-STAT, KIT, and NOTCH1 membrane molecules in promoting tumor growth. Human papilloma virus (HPV) seems to inactivate RB, leading to disruption of cell cycling. P53 and BRCA2 alterations suggest a role of DNA damaging agents. The VEGF pathway and programmed death receptor 1 (PD-1)/PD-ligand (PD-L1) axis also seem to be potentially actionable therapeutic targets.

barrier toward functional validation of these potential therapeutic targets.

NOVEL SYSTEMIC REGIMENS
Targeted Therapies

Epidermal growth factor receptor inhibitors

Overexpression of EGFR has been implicated in the poor prognosis of multiple cancers and is a well-established target for anticancer therapy.[54] Primary PSCC and metastases highly express epidermal growth factor receptor (EGFR) protein.[55–58] In a study of 112 patients, high EGFR expressed by immunohistochemistry (IHC) was noted in 44% of patients and was not associated with grade, histologic subtype, or HPV status.[58] Other smaller studies also corroborate overexpression of EGFR in up to 91% of patients.[47–50,59] Furthermore, KRAS gene mutations, which are associated with resistance to EGFR inhibition, appear infrequent in PSCC, again supporting a potentially major role for EGFR inhibitors in PSCC.[60] Stankiewicz and colleagues[61] analyzed 148 PSCC tumors by IHC and showed that EGFR, HER3, and HER4 but not HER2 was associated with penile carcinogenesis. HPV-negative PSCC expressed more phosphorylated EGFR than HPV-positive PSCC. On the other hand, HER3 expression was more common in HPV-positive PSCC and positively correlated with cytoplasmic Akt expression. This study provides a rationale of targeting HER receptors in PSCC.[61]

Carthon and colleagues[62] retrospectively evaluated the safety and efficacy of EGFR-targeted therapy in 24 patients with advanced PSCC; TTP, OS, responses, and toxicity were studied. All patients had been moderately pretreated, with 22 of 24 patients (91.7%) receiving at least 1 line of prior therapy and 8 of 24 (33.3%) receiving at least 2 lines of prior therapy. Eight patients had received an EGFR-targeted agent alone (cetuximab, erlotinib, or gefitinib); 13 had received cetuximab plus a platinum drug (cisplatin [n = 12] or carboplatin [n = 1]); and 3 patients had received paclitaxel, ifosfamide, cisplatin (TIP) plus cetuximab. Cetuximab had been given with a loading dose of 400 mg/m^2 on day 1 and then at 250 mg/m^2 weekly; erlotinib was given at a dosage of 150 mg orally daily and gefitinib at 250 mg orally daily. The EGFR-targeted therapies were well tolerated; a grade 1 and 2 rash was the most common side effect, occurring in 17 of 24 (70.8%) patients. Grade 3 (severe) or 4 (life-threatening) adverse events that occurred after cetuximab were cellulitis, thrombocytopenia, and bronchospasm in one patient one additional patient's tumor hemorrhaged after cetuximab treatment, which was not thought to be related to therapy.[62] Patients were followed for a median of 207 days; the overall medial TTP was 11.3 weeks, and the median OS was 29.6 weeks. The presence of visceral metastases at the start of anti-EGFR therapy was associated with poor TTP and OS.[62] Partial responses were seen in 1 of 5 patients (20%) who received cetuximab alone, in 3 of 12 patients (25%) who received cetuximab and cisplatin, and in 2 of 3 patients who received cetuximab and TIP. There were no objective responses to gefitinib or erlotinib.[62] In a case report, an objective response was seen with the anti-EGFR monoclonal antibody, panitumumab, following progression after prior cisplatin-based combination chemotherapy.[63] In another case series, 2 of 3 patients derived clinical benefit from EGFR monoclonal antibodies: one patient responded to single-agent cetuximab administered for progressive disease after cisplatin-based chemotherapy and remained disease free for 42 months and another patient symptomatically benefited from panitumumab combined with platinum-based chemotherapy given for disease progression on platinum-based chemotherapy.[64] In contrast, a third patient progressed rapidly on cetuximab despite tumor EGFR expression at the protein and transcriptomic levels. Ongoing trials are evaluating anti-EGFR agents, dacomitinib as neoadjuvant therapy and afatinib as salvage therapy (**Table 4**).

Vascular endothelial growth factor inhibitors

The vascular endothelial growth factor (VEGF) receptor is activated by VEGF-A ligand and overexpressed in approximately 50% of PSCC cases.[65] In a small case series, Zhu and colleagues[66] studied 6 patients with advanced PSCC who were treated with VEGF-tyrosine kinase inhibitors, sorafenib or sunitinib, after receiving at least 2 prior chemotherapy regimens. One out of 6 patients showed a partial response, and 4 patients showed stable disease.[66] Serum SCC antigen and tissue microvessel density and Ki-67 levels were measured before and after therapy; in the partial responder, the serum squamous cell carcinoma (SCC) antigen showed a 95% reduction; in the other patient with stable disease, there was reduction in microvessel density and Ki-67 levels. An ongoing phase II study (PAZOPEN, NCT02279576) is evaluating the combination of pazopanib and weekly paclitaxel in patients with advanced PSCC who have progressed on cisplatin-based chemotherapy (see **Table 4**).[67]

Immunotherapy

Active immunotherapy

Active immunotherapy aims to stimulate the immune response against cancer cells and holds

Table 4
Ongoing clinical trials of systemic therapy for penile squamous cell carcinoma

Clinicaltrials.gov Identifier	Phase	Treatment Population	Sample Size	Treatment
NCT02279576	II	Progressive after platinum-based chemotherapy (PAZOPEN)	32	Pazopanib and paclitaxel
NCT02057913	II	Treatment-naïve advanced/metastatic	22	Vinflunine
NCT02014831	II	Treatment-naïve advanced/metastatic	42	TIP with or without cetuximab
NCT01728233	II	Treatment-naïve neoadjuvant	37	Dacomitinib
NCT02541903	II	Progressive disease after prior chemotherapy	27	Afatinib
Pending	II	Progressive disease after prior chemotherapy	35	Pembrolizumab
NCT02721732	II	Post-therapy rare tumors	250 (including all rare tumors)	Pembrolizumab
NCT01585428	II	Progressive HPV-positive PSCC after standard chemotherapy	73 (including other HPV-positive tumors)	Fludarabine, cyclophosphamide, followed by TIL and high-dose IL-2
NCT02280811	II	Progressive HPV-positive PSCC after standard chemotherapy	61 (including other HPV-positive tumors)	Fludarabine, cyclophosphamide, followed by IL-2 and T-cell targeting HPV-16 E6
NCT02379520	I	Progressive HPV-positive PSCC (HESTIA)	24 (including other HPV-positive tumors)	HPV-16/18 E6/E7–specific T lymphocytes
NCT02526316	I	Progressive HPV-positive PSCC (VICORYX-2)	10 (including other HPV-positive tumors)	Cisplatin-based chemotherapy combined with P16-37-63 peptide vaccination

Abbreviations: IL-2, interleukin-2; TIL, tumor-infiltrating lymphocytes; TIP, paclitaxel, ifosfamide, cisplatin.

great potential in solid tumors. It is know that HPV is implicated in a significant subset of PSCC, with HPV subtypes 16 and 18 found in 40% of patients.[68] The association of HPV with PSCC prognosis is unclear.[59,69,70] Correlation of HPV status and histologic grade of PSCC was reported by Cubilla and colleagues,[71] with 6% of grade 1, 21% of grade 2, and 53% of grade 3 tumors being HPV positive. In a case series of 82 patients with PSCC, HPV-positive tumors had a trend toward a decreased rate of metastases compared with HPV-negative tumors.[72] In another study of 171 patients with PSCC, 29% patients were found to be positive for high-risk HPV and had a significant reduction in risk of dying of PSCC.[73] Large-scale, collaborative, multi-institutional studies are required to further elucidate the role of HPV and PSCC prognosis.

The development of HPV vaccines for primary prevention of cervical cancers in young girls has led to an interest in their use for prevention of PSCC in men. There are several active immunotherapy studies currently ongoing in HPV-induced cancers, including PSCC (see **Table 4**). One study is using tumor-infiltrating lymphocytes for patients with metastatic HPV-associated cancers (NCT01585428).[74] The other study, HESTIA (NCT02379520), is exploring the use of HPV-16/18 E6/E7-specific T lymphocytes for relapsed HPV-associated cancers.[74] A third trial is looking at T cells genetically engineered with a T-cell receptor (TCR) immunotherapy targeting HPV-16 E6

(E6 TCR) (NCT02280811).[74] The combination of cisplatin-based chemotherapy with P16-37 to 63 peptide vaccine is being studied in HPV-positive cancers, including PSCC in another ongoing phase 1 trial (VICORYX-2, NCT02526316). The aforementioned trials will augment our understanding of immunologic mechanisms in PSCC, including HPV-positive PSCC, and how these tumors respond to immunotherapy, including HPV-directed immunologic approaches (see **Table 4**).

T-cell checkpoint signaling pathway inhibitors

Immune checkpoint inhibition with programmed death receptor 1 (PD-1) and the PD-ligand (PD-L1) has changed the landscape of cancer immunotherapy for a variety of cancers.[75–77] In particular, PD-1 and PD-ligand (L)-1 inhibitors are highly active in squamous cell carcinomas of the lung and head and neck, which may bode well for its potential benefit in PSCC.[78,79] Exploiting the PD-1/PD-L1 pathway in PSCC is a rational step to improving the outcomes in this orphan disease whereby no advances have been made in therapeutic options so far. The expression of PD-L1 in PSCC was studied using PSCC tumor specimens.[80] Twenty-three samples between primaries and lymph nodes were collected from 19 patients, with 5 of 23 samples (22%) positive for PD-L1 staining. Six samples (26%) were positive for HPV, with 2 of 6 (33%) HPV-positive patients having positive PD-L1 membrane staining. These findings support the use of checkpoint inhibitors as therapeutic options in PSCC. Sonpavde and colleagues[9] are launching a phase 2 trial with pembrolizumab in metastatic PSCC, and this would provide the much-needed insight into the role of checkpoint inhibitors in this disease (see **Table 4**). Another ongoing phase II trial is evaluating pembrolizumab in patients with a broad spectrum of rare tumors, including PSCC (NCT02721732). Notably, PD-L1 expression is not required for eligibility in both of the aforementioned trials, although tumor tissue will be obtained to evaluate the association of PD-L1 as well as other molecular markers with response.

SUMMARY

PSCC is a rare but lethal disease with current cisplatin-based first-line combination chemotherapy being not curative and second-line therapy offering marginal benefits. The NCCN recommends cisplatin plus 5-fluorouracil or ITP as first-line chemotherapy and paclitaxel or cetuximab as second-line therapy, although trials are highly encouraged. Because of the rarity of the disease, lack of large prospective trials, and absence of

preclinical systems to investigate promising agents, there have been no advances in this orphan disease; incorporation of novel treatment strategies using targeted therapies and immunotherapies is urgently needed to improve outcomes in PSCC. Moreover, the molecular heterogeneity of the disease makes drug development particularly challenging. As we try to better understand the biology of this aggressive disease, designing high-quality biomarker-based trials with attempts to better define prognostic and predictive markers is of utmost importance. Potentially, patients with localized disease proceeding to definitive up-front surgery may be considered for window-of-opportunity trials to identify a signal of biological activity of new agents, as monotherapy or in combination with chemotherapy. Standardization of available therapies as well as developing multi-institutional collaborations, including tissue banking, is imperative to promoting biomarker-driven research across countries. Long-term registries would be a rational step toward lowering the morbidity and mortality in this disease. Regulatory agencies should consider approving drugs based on meeting a threshold of activity in nonrandomized phase II trials enrolling select populations. Greater engagement by the pharmaceutical industry and advocacy groups is critically important to drive drug development for this orphan disease.

There has been some progress in exploring the EGFR- and VEGF-directed therapies in PSCC as single agents or in combination with chemotherapy agents, and results from ongoing prospective trials would provide more insight on the role of targeted therapies. Ongoing immunotherapy trials with vaccines and modified T cells would provide a clearer understanding of the immunology of PSCC and future directions with such therapies. Furthermore, planned trials with checkpoint PD-1 inhibitors that have changed the treatment paradigm across most solid tumors would be crucial to explore and tap their potential merit in this frequently chemo-refractory disease.

REFERENCES

1. Siegel RL, Miller KD, Jemal A. Cancer statistics, 2016. CA Cancer J Clin 2016;66:7–30.
2. Misra S, Chaturvedi A, Misra NC. Penile carcinoma: a challenge for the developing world. Lancet Oncol 2004;5:240–7.
3. Pow-Sang MR, Ferreira U, Pow-Sang JM, et al. Epidemiology and natural history of penile cancer. Urology 2010;76:S2–6.
4. Moses KA, Winer A, Sfakianos JP, et al. Contemporary management of penile cancer: greater than

15 year MSKCC experience. Can J Urol 2014;21: 7201–6.

5. Horenblas S. Lymphadenectomy for squamous cell carcinoma of the penis. Part 1: diagnosis of lymph node metastasis. BJU Int 2001;88:467–72.

6. Spiess PE, National Comprehensive Cancer Network. New treatment guidelines for penile cancer. J Natl Compr Canc Netw 2013;11:659–62.

7. Lopes A, Hidalgo GS, Kowalski LP, et al. Prognostic factors in carcinoma of the penis: multivariate analysis of 145 patients treated with amputation and lymphadenectomy. J Urol 1996;156:1637–42.

8. Protzel C, Ruppin S, Milerski S, et al. The current state of the art of chemotherapy of penile cancer: results of a nationwide survey of German clinics. Urologe A 2009;48:1495–8 [in German].

9. Sonpavde G, Pagliaro LC, Buonerba C, et al. Penile cancer: current therapy and future directions. Ann Oncol 2013;24:1179–89.

10. Di Lorenzo G, Federico P, Buonerba C, et al. Paclitaxel in pretreated metastatic penile cancer: final results of a phase 2 study. Eur Urol 2011; 60:1280–4.

11. Gagliano RG, Blumenstein BA, Crawford ED, et al. Cis-diamminedichloroplatinum in the treatment of advanced epidermoid carcinoma of the penis: a Southwest Oncology Group Study. J Urol 1989; 141:66–7.

12. Ahmed T, Sklaroff R, Yagoda A. An appraisal of the efficacy of bleomycin in epidermoid carcinoma of the penis. Anticancer Res 1984;4:289–92.

13. Sklaroff RB, Yagoda A. Cis-diamminedichloride platinum II (DDP) in the treatment of penile carcinoma. Cancer 1979;44:1563–5.

14. Ahmed T, Sklaroff R, Yagoda A. Sequential trials of methotrexate, cisplatin and bleomycin for penile cancer. J Urol 1984;132:465–8.

15. Garnick MB, Skarin AT, Steele GD Jr. Metastatic carcinoma of the penis: complete remission after high dose methotrexate chemotherapy. J Urol 1979;122:265–6.

16. Shammas FV, Ous S, Fossa SD. Cisplatin and 5-fluorouracil in advanced cancer of the penis. J Urol 1992;147:630–2.

17. Di Lorenzo G, Buonerba C, Federico P, et al. Cisplatin and 5-fluorouracil in inoperable, stage IV squamous cell carcinoma of the penis. BJU Int 2012;110:E661–6.

18. Kattan J, Culine S, Droz JP, et al. Penile cancer chemotherapy: twelve years' experience at Institut Gustave-Roussy. Urology 1993;42:559–62.

19. Theodore C, Skoneczna I, Bodrogi I, et al. A phase II multicentre study of irinotecan (CPT 11) in combination with cisplatin (CDDP) in metastatic or locally advanced penile carcinoma (EORTC PROTOCOL 30992). Ann Oncol 2008;19:1304–7.

20. Joerger M, Warzinek T, Klaeser B, et al. Major tumor regression after paclitaxel and carboplatin polychemotherapy in a patient with advanced penile cancer. Urology 2004;63:778–80.

21. Houede N, Dupuy L, Flechon A, et al. Intermediate analysis of a phase II trial assessing gemcitabine and cisplatin in locoregional or metastatic penile squamous cell carcinoma. BJU Int 2016; 117:444–9.

22. Power DG, Galvin DJ, Cuffe S, et al. Cisplatin and gemcitabine in the management of metastatic penile cancer. Urol Oncol 2009;27:187–90.

23. Dexeus FH, Logothetis CJ, Sella A, et al. Combination chemotherapy with methotrexate, bleomycin and cisplatin for advanced squamous cell carcinoma of the male genital tract. J Urol 1991;146:1284–7.

24. Haas GP, Blumenstein BA, Gagliano RG, et al. Cisplatin, methotrexate and bleomycin for the treatment of carcinoma of the penis: a Southwest Oncology Group study. J Urol 1999;161:1823–5.

25. Hakenberg OW, Nippgen JB, Froehner M, et al. Cisplatin, methotrexate and bleomycin for treating advanced penile carcinoma. BJU Int 2006;98: 1225–7.

26. Corral DA, Sella A, Pettaway CA, et al. Combination chemotherapy for metastatic or locally advanced genitourinary squamous cell carcinoma: a phase II study of methotrexate, cisplatin and bleomycin. J Urol 1998;160:1770–4.

27. Leijte JA, Kerst JM, Bais E, et al. Neoadjuvant chemotherapy in advanced penile carcinoma. Eur Urol 2007;52:488–94.

28. Nicholson S, Hall E, Harland SJ, et al. Phase II trial of docetaxel, cisplatin and 5FU chemotherapy in locally advanced and metastatic penis cancer (CRUK/09/001). Br J Cancer 2013;109:2554–9.

29. Pond GR, Di Lorenzo G, Necchi A, et al. Prognostic risk stratification derived from individual patient level data for men with advanced penile squamous cell carcinoma receiving first-line systemic therapy. Urol Oncol 2014;32(4):501–8.

30. Aparicio LM, Pulido EG, Gallego GA. Vinflunine: a new vision that may translate into antiangiogenic and antimetastatic activity. Anticancer Drugs 2012; 23:1–11.

31. Bermejo C, Busby JE, Spiess PE, et al. Neoadjuvant chemotherapy followed by aggressive surgical consolidation for metastatic penile squamous cell carcinoma. J Urol 2007;177:1335–8.

32. Pizzocaro G, Piva L. Adjuvant and neoadjuvant vincristine, bleomycin, and methotrexate for inguinal metastases from squamous cell carcinoma of the penis. Acta Oncol 1988;27:823–4.

33. Pagliaro LC, Williams DL, Daliani D, et al. Neoadjuvant paclitaxel, ifosfamide, and cisplatin chemotherapy for metastatic penile cancer: a phase II study. J Clin Oncol 2010;28:3851–7.

34. Dickstein RJ, Munsell MF, Pagliaro LC, et al. Prognostic factors influencing survival from regionally

advanced squamous cell carcinoma of the penis after preoperative chemotherapy. BJU Int 2016;117: 118–25.

35. Pizzocaro G, Piva L, Bandieramonte G, et al. Up-to-date management of carcinoma of the penis. Eur Urol 1997;32:5–15.

36. Noronha V, Patil V, Ostwal V, et al. Role of paclitaxel and platinum-based adjuvant chemotherapy in high-risk penile cancer. Urol Ann 2012;4:150–3.

37. O'Reilly A, O'Keeffe M, Aherne P, et al. Treatment of metastatic penile cancer in the adjuvant setting with ifosfamide, paclitaxel, and cisplatin: a single institution experience. J Clin Oncol 2013;31(Suppl 6) [abstract: 340].

38. Hakenberg OW, Comperat EM, Minhas S, et al. EAU guidelines on penile cancer: 2014 update. Eur Urol 2015;67:142–50.

39. Clark PE, Spiess PE, Agarwal N, et al. Penile cancer: clinical practice guidelines in oncology. J Natl Compr Canc Netw 2013;11:594–615.

40. Van Poppel H, Watkin NA, Osanto S, et al. Penile cancer: ESMO clinical practice guidelines for diagnosis, treatment and follow-up. Ann Oncol 2013; 24(Suppl 6):vi115–24.

41. Heideman DA, Waterboer T, Pawlita M, et al. Human papillomavirus-16 is the predominant type etiologically involved in penile squamous cell carcinoma. J Clin Oncol 2007;25:4550–6.

42. Maden C, Sherman KJ, Beckmann AM, et al. History of circumcision, medical conditions, and sexual activity and risk of penile cancer. J Natl Cancer Inst 1993;85:19–24.

43. Hellberg D, Valentin J, Eklund T, et al. Penile cancer: is there an epidemiological role for smoking and sexual behaviour? Br Med J (Clin Res Ed) 1987; 295:1306–8.

44. Gregoire L, Cubilla AL, Reuter VE, et al. Preferential association of human papillomavirus with high-grade histologic variants of penile-invasive squamous cell carcinoma. J Natl Cancer Inst 1995;87:1705–9.

45. Kayes O, Ahmed HU, Arya M, et al. Molecular and genetic pathways in penile cancer. Lancet Oncol 2007;8:420–9.

46. Kayes OJ, Loddo M, Patel N, et al. DNA replication licensing factors and aneuploidy are linked to tumor cell cycle state and clinical outcome in penile carcinoma. Clin Cancer Res 2009;15:7335–44.

47. Bamford S, Dawson E, Forbes S, et al. The COSMIC (catalogue of somatic mutations in cancer) database and website. Br J Cancer 2004;91:355–8. Available at: http://www.sanger.ac.uk/cosmic. Accessed April 17, 2016.

48. Stankiewicz E, Prowse DM, Ktori E, et al. The retinoblastoma protein/p16 INK4A pathway but not p53 is disrupted by human papillomavirus in penile squamous cell carcinoma. Histopathology 2011;58:433–9.

49. McDaniel AS, Hovelson DH, Cani AK, et al. Genomic profiling of penile squamous cell carcinoma reveals new opportunities for targeted therapy. Cancer Res 2015;75:5219–27.

50. Ali SM, Pal SK, Wang K, et al. Comprehensive genomic profiling of advanced penile carcinoma suggests a high frequency of clinically relevant genomic alterations. Oncologist 2016;21:33–9.

51. Naik G, Chen D, Crowley M, et al. Whole-exome sequencing (WES) of penile squamous cell carcinoma (PSCC) to identify multiple recurrent mutations. J Clin Oncol 2016;34(Suppl 2S) [abstract: 484].

52. Mehta AN, Yang ES, Willey CD, et al. Multiplatform comprehensive kinase analysis of penile squamous cell carcinoma (PSCC) to identify drivers and potentially actionable therapeutic targets. J Clin Oncol 2015;33(Suppl 7) [abstract: 389].

53. Mehta AN, Yang ES, Necchi A, et al. Gene expression profiling to improve prognostic stratification of men with advanced penile squamous cell cancer (PSCC) receiving first-line systemic therapy. J Clin Oncol 2015;33(Suppl) [abstract: e15633].

54. Pedersen MW, Meltorn M, Damstrup L, et al. The type III epidermal growth factor receptor mutation. Biological significance and potential target for anti-cancer therapy. Ann Oncol 2001;12:745–60.

55. Lavens N, Gupta R, Wood LA. EGFR overexpression in squamous cell carcinoma of the penis. Curr Oncol 2010;17:4–6.

56. Borgermann C, Schmitz KJ, Sommer S, et al. Characterization of the EGF receptor status in penile cancer: retrospective analysis of the course of the disease in 45 patients. Urologe A 2009;48:1483–9 [in German].

57. Di Lorenzo G, Buonerba C, Ferro M, et al. The epidermal growth factor receptors as biological targets in penile cancer. Expert Opin Biol Ther 2015; 15:473–6.

58. Chaux A, Munari E, Katz B, et al. The epidermal growth factor receptor is frequently overexpressed in penile squamous cell carcinomas: a tissue microarray and digital image analysis study of 112 cases. Hum Pathol 2013;44:2690–5.

59. Agarwal G, Gupta S, Spiess PE. Novel targeted therapies for the treatment of penile cancer. Expert Opin Drug Discov 2014;9:959–68.

60. Gou HF, Li X, Qiu M, et al. Epidermal growth factor receptor (EGFR)-RAS signaling pathway in penile squamous cell carcinoma. PLoS One 2013;8: e62175.

61. Stankiewicz E, Prowse DM, Ng M, et al. Alternative HER/PTEN/Akt pathway activation in HPV positive and negative penile carcinomas. PLoS One 2011; 6:e17517.

62. Carthon BC, Ng CS, Pettaway CA, et al. Epidermal growth factor receptor-targeted therapy in locally

advanced or metastatic squamous cell carcinoma of the penis. BJU Int 2014;113:871–7.

63. Necchi A, Nicolai N, Colecchia M, et al. Proof of activity of anti-epidermal growth factor receptor-targeted therapy for relapsed squamous cell carcinoma of the penis. J Clin Oncol 2011;29:e650–2.

64. Brown A, Ma Y, Danenberg K, et al. Epidermal growth factor receptor-targeted therapy in squamous cell carcinoma of the penis: a report of 3 cases. Urology 2014;83:159–65.

65. Li D, Han Z, Liu J, et al. Upregulation of nucleus HDGF predicts poor prognostic outcome in patients with penile squamous cell carcinoma bypass VEGF-A and Ki-67. Med Oncol 2013;30:702.

66. Zhu Y, Li H, Yao XD, et al. Feasibility and activity of sorafenib and sunitinib in advanced penile cancer: a preliminary report. Urol Int 2010;85:334–40.

67. Climent MA, Puente J, Vazquez-Estevez S, et al. Phase II study of pazopanib and weekly paclitaxel in metastatic or locally advanced squamous penile carcinoma patients previously treated with cisplatin-based chemotherapy: PAZOPEN study. J Clin Oncol 2015;33(Suppl) [abstract: TPS4584].

68. Flaherty A, Kim T, Giuliano A, et al. Implications for human papillomavirus in penile cancer. Urol Oncol 2014;32(53):e51–8.

69. Zhai JP, Wang JW, Man LB. Penile cancer and human papillomavirus infection. Zhonghua Nan Ke Xue 2013;19:178–81 [in Chinese].

70. Zhai JP, Wang QY, Wei D, et al. Association between HPV DNA and disease specific survival in patients with penile cancer. Zhonghua Yi Xue Za Zhi 2013; 93:2719–22 [in Chinese].

71. Cubilla AL, Lloveras B, Alejo M, et al. The basaloid cell is the best tissue marker for human papillomavirus in invasive penile squamous cell carcinoma: a study of 202 cases from Paraguay. Am J Surg Pathol 2010;34:104–14.

72. Bezerra AL, Lopes A, Santiago GH, et al. Human papillomavirus as a prognostic factor in carcinoma of the penis: analysis of 82 patients treated with amputation and bilateral lymphadenectomy. Cancer 2001;91:2315–21.

73. Lont AP, Kroon BK, Horenblas S, et al. Presence of high-risk human papillomavirus DNA in penile carcinoma predicts favorable outcome in survival. Int J Cancer 2006;119:1078–81.

74. Yang JC, Sherry RM, Steinberg SM, et al. Randomized study of high-dose and low-dose interleukin-2 in patients with metastatic renal cancer. J Clin Oncol 2003;21:3127–32.

75. Brahmer JR, Tykodi SS, Chow LQ, et al. Safety and activity of anti-PD-L1 antibody in patients with advanced cancer. N Engl J Med 2012;366:2455–65.

76. Topalian SL, Drake CG, Pardoll DM. Targeting the PD-1/B7-H1(PD-L1) pathway to activate anti-tumor immunity. Curr Opin Immunol 2012;24:207–12.

77. Topalian SL, Hodi FS, Brahmer JR, et al. Safety, activity, and immune correlates of anti-PD-1 antibody in cancer. N Engl J Med 2012;366:2443–54.

78. Seiwert T, Burtness B, Weiss J, et al. A phase Ib study of MK-3475 in patients with human papillomavirus (HPV)-associated and non-HPV–associated head and neck (H/N) cancer. J Clin Oncol 2014; 32(Suppl 5) [abstract: 6011].

79. Segal NH, Antonia SJ, Brahmer JR, et al. Preliminary data from a multi-arm expansion study of MEDI4736, an anti-PD-L1 antibody. J Clin Oncol 2014;32(Suppl 5) [abstract: 3002].

80. Wang J, Rodrigues J, Rao P, et al. Programmed death ligand-1 (PD-L1) expression in penile squamous cell carcinoma. J Clin Oncol 2015;33(Suppl 7) [abstract: 393].

81. Pizzocaro G, Nicolai N, Milani A. Taxanes in combination with cisplatin and fluorouracil for advanced penile cancer: preliminary results. Eur Urol 2009; 55:546–51.

Contemporary Management of Primary Distal Urethral Cancer

 CrossMark

Samer L. Traboulsi, MD[a], Johannes Alfred Witjes, MD, PhD[b],
Wassim Kassouf, MD, CM, FRCS(C)[a],*

KEYWORDS

- Urethra • Urethral neoplasms • Therapeutics • Therapy

KEY POINTS

- Stage and anatomic location of the primary urethral tumor guide the choice of treatment modality and are the main determinants of prognosis and survival.
- Surgical options range from local excision to transurethral resection to partial urethrectomy/penectomy to total penectomy in men or excision of the urethra, vulva, and vaginal wall in women.
- For distal urethral tumors, surgical options are more appropriate for men whereas radiation therapy is a reasonable option in women.
- Routine inguinal or ilioinguinal lymphadenectomy for higher-stage tumors should be considered; however, there are few data derived from the treatment of primary urethral cancer to support it.
- Multimodal therapy is usually reserved for more advanced stages in combination with surgery to improve survival.

INTRODUCTION

Epidemiology

Primary urethral carcinomas (PUCs) are rare and account for less than 1% of genitourinary cancers.[1,2] Most of the data rely on studies with small numbers of patients or case reports. PUCs arise from the urethral epithelium or from periurethral glands.[3,4] The incidence of PUCs is known to be 3 to 4 times more common in women than in men. Recent data from the Surveillance, Epidemiology, and End Results (SEER) database, however, reported higher incidence in men, with an annual age-adjusted incidence rate of PUCs of 4.3 per million in men and 1.5 per million in women.[5]

Etiology

Chronic inflammation, strictures, and sexually transmitted diseases are implicated in PUC.

Columnar and mucinous adenocarcinoma may arise from glandular metaplasia and cribriform adenocarcinoma has its origins from the prostate.[6] Squamous cell carcinoma (SCC) is associated with human papillomavirus (HPV) infection in both genders. HPV 16 or HPV 18 is associated in 60% of urethral carcinoma in women[7] and HPV 16 is associated with 30% of pendulous urethra SCC in men.[8,9] More than half the patients diagnosed with PUC have a history of stricture, and 25% have a history of sexually transmitted disease.[2]

Anatomic Histopathology

In men, the anterior urethra includes the penile and the bulbous urethra. The posterior urethra includes the prostatic and the membranous urethra. In women, the anterior urethra constitutes

The authors declare no commercial or financial conflicts of interest.
[a] Department of Urology, McGill University Health Centre, 1001 Decarie Boulevard, Montreal, Quebec H4A3J1, Canada; [b] Department of Urology, Radboud University Nijmegen Medical Centre, Geert Grooteplein South 10 (659), PO Box 9101, 6500 HB Nijmegen, The Netherlands
* Corresponding author. McGill University Health Centre, Glen Site D02.7210, 1001 Decarie Boulevard, Montreal, Quebec H4A 3J1, Canada.
E-mail address: wassim.kassouf@muhc.mcgill.ca

Urol Clin N Am 43 (2016) 493–503
http://dx.doi.org/10.1016/j.ucl.2016.06.010
0094-0143/16/© 2016 Elsevier Inc. All rights reserved.

urologic.theclinics.com

the distal one-third whereas the proximal two-thirds constitute the posterior urethra.[10] The distal urethra in men is the penile and glandular urethra whereas in women the distal urethra constitutes the distal one-third of the urethra.[11]

In women, lymphatics from the posterior urethra drain to the external and internal iliac and obturator lymph node chains. The anterior urethra drains to the superficial and then to the deep inguinal lymph nodes. In men, the lymphatics from the anterior urethra drain into the superficial and deep inguinal lymph nodes (and occasionally into the external iliac lymph nodes). The posterior urethra drains directly into one or any combination of the presacral, obturator, and external iliac lymphatic channels.[12,13]

Different histologic types for PUC follow an anatomic distribution due to the presence of different epithelial histology depending on location (**Fig. 1**). SCC is believed the most common type, representing more than 60% of PUCs in men and women. According to contemporary data extracted from the SEER, however, the distribution may be different. Among women, urothelial carcinoma (UC), SCC, and adenocarcinoma each represented approximately 30% of PUCs.[5] In men, UC represented 78%, SCC 12% and adenocarcinoma 5% of cases.[14]

PATIENT EVALUATION OVERVIEW
Clinical Presentation

PUCs can present with hematuria or bloody urethral discharge. These are the presenting symptoms in up to 62% of the cases. Symptoms of locally advanced disease include a palpable urethral mass in 52%, bladder outlet obstruction in 48%, pelvic pain in 33%, urethrocutaneous fistula in 10%, and abscess formation in 5%.[15] When they become clinically evident, urethral cancers are already locally advanced in 45% to 57%[15,16]

Clinical Evaluation

For local staging, clinical examination should include palpation of the external genitalia and digital rectal examination in men to assess for mass/induration. In women, palpation of the urethra should be done. Speculum visualization to inspect the vaginal wall and vulva is also advised, in addition to bimanual examination. Palpation of the inguinal lymph nodes should be routinely performed.[17,18] In contrast to penile cancer, the presence of palpable lymph nodes in urethral cancer is almost always metastasis.[8,19–21]

Urine Cytology

The sensitivity of urine cytology in detecting PUC varies according to gender and histologic type. In a study by Toujier and Dalbagni,[22] the sensitivity

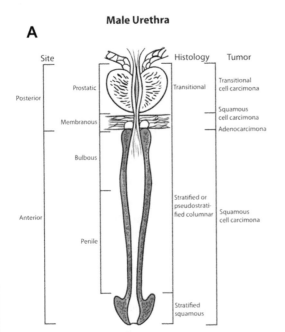

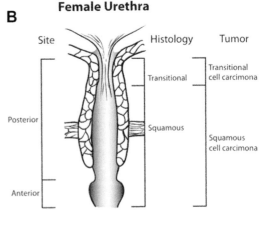

Fig. 1. Anatomic distribution of histologic types and corresponding histopathology in male (*A*) and female (*B*) urethra. (*Adapted from* Sharp DS, Angermeier KW. Tumors of the urethra [Fig. 38.1 and 38.9]. In: Wein AJ, Kavoussi LR, Partin AW, editors. Campbell-Walsh urology. 11th edition. Philadelphia: Elsevier; 2016. p. 880, 886; with permission.)

of urine cytology for UC in men was 80% compared with 50% in women. For SCC, however, the sensitivity in men was 50% compared with 77% in women.

Urethrocystoscopy

Urethroscopy and biopsy visualize the urethral tumor appearance, location, and extent and determine the histologic type.[18] A concomitant cystoscopy should be performed to rule out the presence of a concomitant primary bladder tumor.[23]

Imaging

Radiologic imaging is used to assess local tumor spread and metastasis to lymph nodes and distal organs. MRI is an excellent modality for local tumor staging of PUC (**Tables 1** and **2**). MRI can assess involvement of the corpora cavernosa, status of pelvic and inguinal lymph nodes, and response to chemotherapy.[24–27] The accuracy of MRI for staging urethral cancer has been reported to be approximately 75% and is superior to CT in visualizing tissue planes.[28]

Table 1
Tumor staging

Primary urethral (male and female)	
TX	Primary tumor cannot be assessed
T0	No evidence of primary tumor
Ta	Noninvasive papillary, polypoid, or verrucous carcinoma
Tis	CIS
Tis pu	CIS, involvement of prostatic urethra
Tis pd	CIS, involvement of prostatic ducts
T1	Tumor invades subepithelial connective tissue
T2	Tumor invades any of the following: corpus spongiosum, prostatic stroma, periurethral muscle
T3	Tumor invades any of the following: corpus cavernosum, beyond prostatic capsule, anterior vagina, bladder neck (extraprostatic extension)
T4	Tumor invades other adjacent organs
Regional lymph nodes	
NX	Regional lymph nodes cannot be assessed
N0	No regional lymph node metastasis
N1	Metastasis in a single lymph node 2 cm or less in greatest dimension
N2	Metastasis in a single lymph node more than 2 cm in greatest dimension or multiple lymph nodes
Distant metastasis	
MX	Distant metastasis cannot be assessed
M0	No distant metastasis
M1	Distant metastasis
Histopathologic grading (urothelial)	
PUNLUMP	Papillary urothelial neoplasm of low malignant potential
Low-grade	Well differentiated
High-grade	Poorly differentiated
Histopathologic grading (nonurothelial)	
GX	Grade of differentiation cannot be assessed
G1	Well differentiated
G2	Moderately differentiated
G3-4	Poorly differentiated/undifferentiated

From Sobin LH, Gospodarowicz MK, Wittekind C, editors. TNM classification of malignant tumors. UICC International Union Against Cancer. 7th edition. Wiley-Blackwell; 2009.

Table 2
Stage grouping

Stage Grouping			
Stage 0a	Ta	N0	M0
Stage 0is	Tis	N0	M0
	Tis pu	N0	M0
	Tis pd	N0	Mo
Stage I	T1	N0	M0
Stage II	T2	N0	M0
Stage III	T1/T2	N1	M0
	T3	N0/N1	M0
Stage IV	T4	N0/N1	M0
	Any T	N2	M0
	Any T	Any N	M1

From Sobin LH, Gospodarowicz MK, Wittekind C, editors. TNM classification of malignant tumors. UICC International Union Against Cancer. 7th edition. Wiley-Blackwell; 2009.

CT scan of the abdomen, in addition to chest radiograph (or CT chest) should be performed in all patients with invasive disease to detect distant metastases. PET CT is a promising modality for the detection of lymph node involvement and distant metastasis for PUC. PET CT is particularly useful for looking at suspicious sites of metastasis detected on alternate imaging (ie, CT/MRI).[29]

PHARMACOLOGIC TREATMENT OPTIONS

One report discusses successful treatment with topical fluorouracil (5-FU) cream of carcinoma in situ (CIS) located close to or at the meatal opening in 2 patients.[30] After treatment, 1 patient had no evidence of disease at 13 months and the other was also disease-free at 26 months.

SURGICAL TREATMENT OPTIONS IN MEN

The standard treatment of distal PUC is total or partial penectomy. The surgical approach in PUC is derived from surgery for penile carcinoma. The size, stage, and anatomic location of a distal PUC dictate the choice of the surgical approach. A partial penectomy is chosen when residual penile length is sufficient with negative surgical margins. In urethral cancer, the traditional excision margin of 2 cm has been extrapolated from the general traditional management of penile carcinoma.[31] Recent reports in penile cancer suggest that margins can be limited to 1 cm without compromising oncologic control.[31,32] Furthermore, a large series on primary distal urethral

cancer in men has achieved excellent local disease control even with margins less than 5 mm.[30] Other more conservative penile-preserving approaches, such as transurethral resection, partial urethrectomy, and radiation, have been reported with satisfactory results in select cases.

Dinney and colleagues[33] reported on 15 men with tumors in the penile urethra (n = 11) or fossa navicularis (n = 4) treated primarily with surgery. Tumors of the fossa navicularis of all stages were treated with either partial urethrectomy or partial penectomy with disease-specific survival (DSS) rates of 100% after a mean follow-up of 93 months. Penile urethral cancers had a DSS of 60% after a mean follow-up of 48 (5–156) months. Treatment consisted of surgical monotherapy in 5, a combination of surgery and chemotherapy in 4, and chemotherapy alone in 2. Surgical monotherapy consisted of 3 partial penectomies, 1 total penectomy with cystoprostatectomy, and 1 partial penectomy with pelvic node dissection. Two patients required adjuvant chemotherapy after surgery due to the presence of positive sentinel node biopsy.

Penile-preserving surgery, such as transurethral fulguration, local excision, or partial urethrectomy, is an attractive alternative to the traditional penectomy approach for early-stage distal tumors. The efficacy of these penile-preserving approaches in achieving long-term disease-free survival has been demonstrated by several studies (**Table 3**). A series from the United Kingdom reported on penile-preserving surgeries for 18 men with distal PUC.[30] Within a mean follow-up of 26 (9–58) months, 78% of the patients were alive and free of disease. One patient with a T1 tumor and 2 patients with CIS of the meatus were treated with biopsy and formation of hypospadias followed by topical 5-FU cream. Four patients underwent a 2-stage urethroplasty with buccal mucosa flap and 3 were treated with glansectomy with hypospadias and partial-thickness skin graft reconstruction. Six patients were treated with partial penectomy and reconstruction and 2 patients with large tumors of the penile urethra underwent anterior urethrectomy and perineal urethrostomy.

Glans-preserving surgery has been described to improve the esthetics and lessen the psychological trauma of dismemberment and emasculation. Bird and Coburn[34] reported on a glans-preserving technique in 2 patients with T2 and T3 distal urethral SCC. The technique consisted of a subcutaneous penectomy achieved by resection of the urethra and corpora cavernosae with preservation of the penile skin and the glans for subsequent phallic reconstruction. No patient developed

Table 3
Results of conservative surgery in male patients with distal urethral tumors

Author	Patients (n)	Stage	Treatment (n)	Outcome
Mandler & Pool,[35] 1966	3	—	Fulguration/excision	NED 2–20 y
Konnak,[36] 1980	8	—	Excision	NED 1–13 y
Bracken et al,[37] 1980	1	—	Excision	NED 236 mo
Gheiler et al,[15] 1998	4	T1-T2	• Transurethral resection (1) • Distal urethrectomy (1) • Distal urethrectomy + inguinal dissection (1); • Neoadjuvant chemoradiation + partial urethrectomy	• NED 61 mo • NED 36 mo • NED 37 mo • NED 36 mo
Dinney et al,[33] 1994	1	T1	Distal urethrectomy	NED 152 mo
Smith et al,[30] 2007	7	CIS, T1, T2	• Excision (3) • Two-stage distal urethroplasty with BCM flap (4)	• NED 13–36 mo • NED 13–47 mo

Abbreviations: BCM, buccal mucosa; NED, no evidence of disease.

local recurrence at 22 months' follow-up; however, distant metastases did occur in both patients.

RADIATION THERAPY IN MEN

Reports on radiation monotherapy in male distal PUCs are scarce and the results generally not encouraging. Bracken and colleagues[37] reported on 11 patients with penile urethra tumors, treated surgically in 9 cases and with radiation monotherapy in 2 cases. Those treated with radiation monotherapy died of their disease at 7 and 30 months. Hopkins and colleagues[38] reported on 1 patient with SCC of the pendulous urethra with positive inguinal lymph nodes treated with 30 Gy of radiation in addition to inguinal node dissection. This patient developed lung metastases 7 months later and died at 22 months. Raghaviah reported on 2 patients with penile urethral carcinoma treated with 50 Gy to 55 Gy external beam radiotherapy (EBRT) who refused amputation.[39] Both patients were alive with no evidence of disease after 4 years.

Overall, the data on radiotherapy as a monotherapy are scant and had not shown promising results in male PUC. Radiation-induced complications, especially urethral strictures, can be significant and difficult to manage.[39–41] Until further studies, radiation therapy should be reserved for patients with early-stage distal disease who refuse surgery.

COMBINATION THERAPIES IN MEN

Distal PUC in men has been successfully treated with surgery as a single modality, especially in low-stage tumors. In higher-stage urethral cancer, the risk of failure (local, nodal, and distal metastasis) is higher. The addition of radiotherapy, chemotherapy, or a combination of both with surgery has been reported in anterior urethral tumors. Gheiler and colleagues[15] reported on a total of 6 patients with T2N0 distal cancers; 3 treated with surgery alone and 3 with combination therapy (2 neoadjuvant chemoradiotherapy and 1 with adjuvant radiotherapy). All patients were disease-free at a mean follow-up of 41 months and 50 months, respectively. In this small series, the results of surgical monotherapy for distal tumors were comparable to combination therapy in low-stage, node negative patients.

The combination of surgery with chemotherapy was successful for more advanced tumors with positive inguinal lymph nodes in the MD Anderson Cancer Center (MDACC) series.[33] Among the 5 patients treated with combination therapy, 4 were alive and disease-free after a median follow-up of 77 months. Baskin and Turzan[42] described a case of T3 distal urethral SCC with palpable right groin lymph nodes who was treated with 5-FU and mitomycin C. Radiotherapy was also given to the primary site, pelvic and inguinal areas followed by distal urethrectomy. The investigators report complete downstaging of the tumor with no evidence of disease on pathology.

Cohen and colleagues[43] reported on 18 cases of PUC involving the pendulous in 9 and the bulbomembranous urethra in 9 cases: 12 patients with T2–4 tumors, 1 with TxN1, and 5 with TxN2 disease. All patients received a protocol of MMC and 5-FU combined with EBRT. Three patients did not respond and eventually died at a mean follow-up of 11.7 months from salvage surgery; 15 patients achieved an initial complete response to the chemoradiation protocol, 10 of whom never recurred with 8 remaining alive with no evidence of disease at mean follow-up of 65 months.

In summary, use of multimodal therapy should be considered in patients with non–organ-confined disease ($\geq$T3 or nodal metastasis). Reports are limited by small sample size of retrospective series treated with varying multimodal protocols.

SURGICAL TREATMENT OPTIONS IN WOMEN

Similar to PUC in men, the prognosis of urethral tumors in women depends on the size, stage, and anatomic location.[1,44,45] Large tumor size is associated with poor prognosis. One study reported 5-year survival for tumors smaller than 2 cm to be 60% compared with 13% for tumors larger than 5 cm.[44] Most of the reports failed to detect a survival difference between the histologic types of PUC with the exception of melanoma.[1,46,47] With those patients receiving partial urethrectomy or radical extirpation for PUC with melanoma histology, the overall and cancer-specific survival rates at 3 years were 27% and 38%, respectively.[47]

Dalbagni and colleagues[1] reported on 72 patients with PUC treated with monotherapy (surgery or radiotherapy) with a 5-year recurrence-free survival of only 46%. When considering distal urethral tumors, these are usually lower stage than tumors of the proximal urethra and associated with improved 5-year metastasis-free survival (71% vs 48%, respectively).[1]

Distal low-stage Ta-T1 tumors at the meatus can be treated with local excision, transurethral resection, or distal urethrectomy with intraoperative frozen sections to ensure negative surgical margins.[45,48] Dimarco and colleagues[48] reported on 29 patients with carcinoma of the distal urethra. There were 17 patients with T1-2 tumors and 5 with T3 tumors who underwent partial urethrectomy; 9 required an additional vulvar or vaginal resection. The remainder of patients (4 with T2 and 3 T3–4 tumors) underwent either anterior pelvic exenteration or radical urethrectomy with bladder preservation. The 5-year DSS for patients with distal tumors was 73%. In this series, there was a local recurrence in 21% of patients with stage T2 that required salvage therapy. The investigators advised a radical urethrectomy with closure of bladder neck and creation of a catheterizable stoma in select patients with T2-3 tumors.[48,49]

RADIATION THERAPY IN WOMEN

According to most studies, women treated with radiation therapy for distal PUC seem to have similar survival outcomes compared with those treated with surgery.[41] In women, radiotherapy is associated with less morbidity compared with surgery. Resection of the distal third of the urethra with adequate surgical margins has an increased risk of sphincteric injury. For low-stage tumors, radiation therapy as single modality seems to be effective for distal PUC (**Table 4**).[50–52]

The MDACC group reported successful local control in all 5 patients with stages I and II PUC after a median follow-up of 4 years; 4 patients received brachytherapy alone and 1 patient received a combination of EBRT and brachytherapy. None of the patients developed recurrence.[50] Prempree and colleagues[53] treated 3 patients with distal urethral cancers with brachytherapy only and reported a 100% local control and 5-year survival. In a retrospective study on 86 women treated either with brachytherapy and/or EBRT, Garden and colleagues[54] found that the method of radiation delivery did not have an impact on outcome; only the urethral length involved with disease was an independent prognostic factor. The 5-year local control rate was 74% for tumors involving part of the urethra versus 48% for tumors involving the entire urethra.

Table 4 Results of radiation only for female primary urethral carcinoma					
Author	Number of Patients	Radiation	Mean Follow-up (mo)	Overall Survival (%)	Local Control (%)
Moinuddin Ali et al,[51] 1988	3	EBRT + BT	27	67	100
Johnson & O'Connell,[50] 1983	5	BT ± EBRT	41	80	60
Prempree et al,[53] 1984	7	BT ± EBRT	—	—	71
Weghaupt et al,[55] 1984	42	Intacavitary RT + EBRT	—	71	—

Abbreviations: BT, brachytherapy; CSM, cause specific mortality; DFS, disease-free survival; RT, radiotherapy.

An older series reported lower rates of local failures in patients treated with radiotherapy compared with surgery alone (36% vs 60%).[46] Combination of brachytherapy and EBRT yielded better control of disease. Another report from Austria included 42 women with anterior tumors, a majority of whom had SCC histology.[55] A radiation dose of 55 Gy to 70 Gy was delivered through a combination of intracavitary vaginal irradiation and EBRT. Large tumors of the anterior urethra underwent transurethral resection before radiation. Palpable lymph nodes were present in 40.5% of patients with distal PUC; most were treated with radiation to the inguinal fields. The 5-year overall survival for distal PUC was 71.4%.

In summary, radiation therapy for distal PUC provides adequate local control and increased survival advantage in women. Early-stage distal tumors can be treated with radiation only. EBRT can be added to brachytherapy in more advanced disease of the distal urethra to include the groin and/or the pelvis.

COMBINATION THERAPIES IN WOMEN

Multimodal therapy is commonly used for posterior PUC or advanced PUC to improve outcomes. Combination therapies have also been reported, however, for distal tumors of the female urethra. Licht and colleagues[56] report a case of stage T3N0M0 SCC of the distal urethra where the patient was treated with a combination of chemoradiotherapy consisting of 5-FU and mitomycin C with EBRT and remained disease-free at 43 months. In another report, Dalbagni and colleagues[57] reported a case of distal urethral UC treated with anterior exenteration with intraoperative brachytherapy followed by EBRT (pT2N0M0). The patient was alive and disease-free at 47 months' follow-up. In a series encompassing locally advanced tumors, radiation therapy delivered prior to surgery resulted in 5-year overall survival rates of 75% and in excellent local control rates.[50,51] Therefore, combination therapies should be considered for non–organ-confined distal PUC to increase local disease control rates.

LYMPH NODES MANAGEMENT

The management of lymph nodes in patients with PUC has not yet been established. In men, tumors of the penile urethra primarily involve the groin nodes whereas tumors of the bulbar urethra usually involve the pelvic nodes.[18] The value of prophylactic lymphadenectomy in the absence of gross lymphadenopathy has not

been demonstrated but ilioinguinal lymphadenectomy is advocated in case of palpable adenopathy. The inguinal lymphadenectomy technique is similar to that used for the treatment of the penile cancer.[58] Dinney and colleagues[33] showed that patients with low-volume nodal disease, performance of lymphadenectomy can achieve disease-free survival up to 156 months. It is unknown, however, whether prolonged survival achieved was a result of lymphadenectomy or the use of adjuvant chemotherapy. With limited data, it is reasonable to advocate prophylactic inguinal nodal dissection for patients with invasive disease (≥T2).

In women, tumors of the distal one-third of the urethra can be accompanied by metastasis to superficial and deep inguinal lymph nodes. Similar to PUC in men, there is no clear evidence that prophylactic lymph node dissection in the absence of gross disease is beneficial.[48] An older report also showed no survival advantage for gross adenopathy treated with pelvic or inguinal lymphadenectomy.[11] Weghaupt and colleagues[55] reported a 71% 5-year survival rate in 42 patients with distal PUC, 40.5% of whom had evidence of lymph node involvement. Patients with lymphadenopathy received radiation to the nodes in most of the cases. In the presence of lymph nodes greater than or equal to 2 cm, however, only 1 of 7 patients survived 5 years.

COMPLICATIONS

Rates of complications have ranged from 20% to 40% and include urinary incontinence, urethral strictures, fistulae formation, cystitis, vulvar abscess, and cellulitis, urethral necrosis, external genitalia necrosis, necrosis of pelvic bones, and bladder or small bowel obstruction.[40,54,59] In women, radiation therapy could also result in fistula formation in tumors invading the vagina.[60] Higher rates of urethral strictures observed after radiation for PUC in men compared with women.[43] Overall, complications have decreased with modern and reduced dose of radiation.[54,60] Ilioinguinal lymph node dissection can also be associated with significant morbidity, especially in women. Weghaupt and colleagues[55] reported a significant risk of death with ilioinguinal lymphadenectomy, especially in older women.

EVALUATION OF OUTCOME AND LONG-TERM RECOMMENDATIONS

In PUC, prognostic factors for recurrence-free survival and overall survival have been identified.

Gakis and colleagues[20] showed that for patients with no distal metastases at diagnosis, recurrence-free survival was significantly associated with clinical nodal stage, tumor location, and age, whereas clinical nodal stage was the only independent predictor for overall survival. Distal tumors are associated with a longer recurrence-free survival compared with proximal tumors (relative risk = 2.33; P = .002). Few data are available for a consensus in the treatment of distal PUC. The general guiding variables, however, for the choice of the treatment modality are the stage, extent, anatomic location of the tumor, and gender.[20] In men, there are several reasons that render surgery the mainstay of therapy for distal PUC. Overall surgical approaches have achieved adequate local control of the disease and satisfactory long-term disease-free survival rates. Furthermore, in select groups of patients, penile-preserving surgeries could be used safely and decrease the psychological burden of dismemberment. Radiotherapy does not achieve comparable local disease control rates compared with surgery. The complications of radiotherapy,

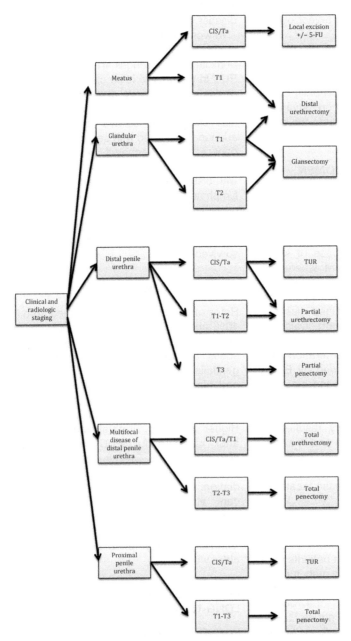

Fig. 2. Management of primary distal urethral carcinoma in men.

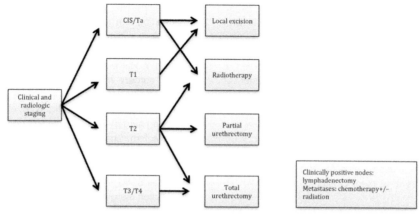

Fig. 3. Management of primary distal urethral carcinoma in women.

especially urethral strictures, are high and difficult to manage.

In women, radiotherapy is generally preferred to surgery in the treatment of distal PUC. Furthermore, due to the short urethral length in women, it is difficult to achieve adequate surgical margins without compromising sphincteric function in women treated with surgical resection. For men and women, inguinal or ilioinguinal lymph node dissection is advocated for clinically positive inguinal lymphadenopathy in the context of multimodal therapy. In cases of pelvic lymphadenopathy, a surgical approach combined with chemotherapy is advocated. The role of prophylactic lymphadenectomy in node-negative disease is unknown. **Figs. 2** and **3** provide an algorithm for the management of distal PUC in men and women.

SUMMARY

PUC is a rare disease. Most of the data available are derived from small case series. Most of the reported treatments for PUC are not standardized and vary between different institutions. The general strategy in the treatment of PUC depends on gender, stage, and location of the tumor. In early-stage distal PUC, the main aim is to achieve an adequate local control of the disease. Organ-preserving approaches are advocated in men if oncologically safe. In women, radiation portray similar outcomes and is commonly used because there can be a high rate of urinary incontinence and sexual dysfunction encountered with surgical resection.

REFERENCES

1. Dalbagni G, Zhang ZF, Lacombe L, et al. Female urethral carcinoma: an analysis of treatment outcome and a plea for a standardized management strategy. Br J Urol 1998;82:835.

2. Dalbagni G, Zhang ZF, Lacombe L, et al. Male urethral carcinoma: analysis of treatment outcome. Urology 1999;53:1126.

3. Amin MB, Young RH. Primary carcinomas of the urethra. Semin Diagn Pathol 1997;14:147.

4. Reis LO, Billis A, Ferreira FT, et al. Female urethral carcinoma: evidences to origin from Skene's glands. Urol Oncol 2011;29:218.

5. Swartz MA, Porter MP, Lin DW, et al. Incidence of primary urethral carcinoma in the United States. Urology 2006;68:1164.

6. Murphy DP, Pantuck AJ, Amenta PS, et al. Female urethral adenocarcinoma: immunohistochemical evidence of more than 1 tissue of origin. J Urol 1881; 161:1999.

7. Wiener JS, Walther PJ. A high association of oncogenic human papillomaviruses with carcinomas of the female urethra: polymerase chain reaction-based analysis of multiple histological types. J Urol 1994;151:49.

8. Cupp MR, Malek RS, Goellner JR, et al. Detection of human papillomavirus DNA in primary squamous cell carcinoma of the male urethra. Urology 1996; 48:551.

9. Wiener JS, Liu ET, Walther PJ. Oncogenic human papillomavirus type 16 is associated with squamous cell cancer of the male urethra. Cancer Res 1992;52: 5018.

10. Sharp DS, Angermeier KW. Tumors of the urethra. In: Wein AJ, Kavoussi LR, Partin AW, et al, editors. Campbell-Walsh urology, vol. 1, 11th edition. Philadelphia: Elsevier; 2016. p. 879–89.

11. Grabstald H. Proceedings: tumors of the urethra in men and women. Cancer 1973;32:1236.

12. Chao KSC, Perez CA. Penis and male urethra. In: Perez CA, Brady LW, editors. Principles and practice of radiation oncology. 3rd edition. Philadelphia: Lippincott-Raven; 1997. p. 1717–31.

13. Gerbaulet A, Haie-Meder C, Marsiglia H, et al. Brachytherapy in cancer of the urethra. Ann Urol (Paris) 1994;28:312 [in French].

14. Rabbani F. Prognostic factors in male urethral cancer. Cancer 2011;117:2426.

15. Gheiler EL, Tefilli MV, Tiguert R, et al. Management of primary urethral cancer. Urology 1998;52:487.

16. Golijanin D, Yossepowitch O, Beck SD, et al. Carcinoma in a bladder diverticulum: presentation and treatment outcome. J Urol 2003;170:1761.

17. Blaivas JG, Flisser AJ, Bleustein CB, et al. Periurethral masses: etiology and diagnosis in a large series of women. Obstet Gynecol 2004;103:842.

18. Karnes RJ, Breau RH, Lightner DJ. Surgery for urethral cancer. Urol Clin North Am 2010;37:445.

19. Dayyani F, Pettaway CA, Kamat AM, et al. Retrospective analysis of survival outcomes and the role of cisplatin-based chemotherapy in patients with urethral carcinomas referred to medical oncologists. Urol Oncol 2013;31:1171.

20. Gakis G, Morgan TM, Efstathiou JA, et al. Prognostic factors and outcomes in primary urethral cancer: results from the international collaboration on primary urethral carcinoma. World J Urol 2016;34:97.

21. Gakis G, Daneshmand S, Efstathiou JA, et al. prognostic factors and outcomes after definitive treatment for primary urethral cancer: results of the international collaboration on primary urethral Carcinoma. J Urol 2013;189(4 Suppl):e388.

22. Touijer AK, Dalbagni G. Role of voided urine cytology in diagnosing primary urethral carcinoma. Urology 2004;63:33.

23. Gakis G, Efstathiou JA, Morgan T, et al. Impact of synchronous bladder cancer on recurrence- free survival after surgical treatment for primary urethral cancer: results of the international Collaboration on Primary Urethral Carcinoma (ICPUC). J Urol 2014; 191(4 Suppl):176–7.

24. Kim B, Kawashima A, LeRoy AJ. Imaging of the male urethra. Semin Ultrasound CT MR 2007;28:258.

25. Lont AP, Besnard AP, Gallee MP, et al. A comparison of physical examination and imaging in determining the extent of primary penile carcinoma. BJU Int 2003;91:493.

26. Ryu J, Kim B. MR imaging of the male and female urethra. Radiographics 2001;21:1169.

27. Gourtsoyianni S, Hudolin T, Sala E, et al. MRI at the completion of chemoradiotherapy can accurately evaluate the extent of disease in women with advanced urethral carcinoma undergoing anterior pelvic exenteration. Clin Radiol 2011;66: 1072.

28. Stewart SB, Leder RA, Inman BA. Imaging tumors of the penis and urethra. Urol Clin North Am 2010; 37:353.

29. Graafland NM, Leijte JA, Valdes Olmos RA, et al. Scanning with 18F-FDG-PET/CT for detection of pelvic nodal involvement in inguinal node-positive penile carcinoma. Eur Urol 2009;56:339.

30. Smith Y, Hadway P, Ahmed S, et al. Penile-preserving surgery for male distal urethral carcinoma. BJU Int 2007;100:82.

31. Hegarty PK, Shabbir M, Hughes B, et al. Penile preserving surgery and surgical strategies to maximize penile form and function in penile cancer: recommendations from the United Kingdom experience. World J Urol 2009;27:179.

32. Minhas S, Kayes O, Hegarty P, et al. What surgical resection margins are required to achieve oncological control in men with primary penile cancer? BJU Int 2005;96:1040.

33. Dinney CP, Johnson DE, Swanson DA, et al. Therapy and prognosis for male anterior urethral carcinoma: an update. Urology 1994;43:506.

34. Bird E, Coburn M. Phallus preservation for urethral cancer: subcutaneous penectomy. J Urol 1997; 158:2146.

35. Mandler JI, Pool TL. Primary carcinoma of the male urethra. J Urol 1966;96:67.

36. Konnak JW. Conservative management of low grade neoplasms of the male urethra: a preliminary report. J Urol 1980;123:175.

37. Bracken RB, Henry R, Ordonez N. Primary carcinoma of the male urethra. South Med J 1980;73: 1003.

38. Hopkins SC, Nag SK, Soloway MS. Primary carcinoma of male urethra. Urology 1984;23:128.

39. Raghavaiah NV. Radiotherapy in the treatment of carcinoma of the male urethra. Cancer 1978;41: 1313.

40. Forman JD, Lichter AS. The role of radiation therapy in the management of carcinoma of the male and female urethra. Urol Clin North Am 1992;19:383.

41. Koontz BF, Lee WR. Carcinoma of the urethra: radiation oncology. Urol Clin North Am 2010;37:459.

42. Baskin LS, Turzan C. Carcinoma of male urethra: management of locally advanced disease with combined chemotherapy, radiotherapy, and penile-preserving surgery. Urology 1992;39:21.

43. Cohen MS, Triaca V, Billmeyer B, et al. Coordinated chemoradiation therapy with genital preservation for the treatment of primary invasive carcinoma of the male urethra. J Urol 2008;179:536.

44. Bracken RB, Johnson DE, Miller LS, et al. Primary carcinoma of the female urethra. J Urol 1976;116:188.

45. Narayan P, Konety B. Surgical treatment of female urethral carcinoma. Urol Clin North Am 1992;19:373.

46. Foens CS, Hussey DH, Staples JJ, et al. A comparison of the roles of surgery and radiation therapy in the management of carcinoma of the female urethra. Int J Radiat Oncol Biol Phys 1991;21:961.

47. DiMarco DS, DiMarco CS, Zincke H, et al. Outcome of surgical treatment for primary malignant melanoma of the female urethra. J Urol 2004;171:765.

48. Dimarco DS, Dimarco CS, Zincke H, et al. Surgical treatment for local control of female urethral carcinoma. Urol Oncol 2004;22:404.

49. Rajan N, Tucci P, Mallouh C, et al. Carcinoma in female urethral diverticulum: case reports and review of management. J Urol 1993;150:1911.

50. Johnson DE, O'Connell JR. Primary carcinoma of female urethra. Urology 1983;21:42.

51. Moinuddin Ali M, Klein FA, Hazra TA. Primary female urethral carcinoma. A retrospective comparison of different treatment techniques. Cancer 1988;62:54.

52. Prempree T, Wizenberg MJ, Scott RM. Radiation treatment of primary carcinoma of the female urethra. Cancer 1978;42:1177.

53. Prempree T, Amornmarn R, Patanaphan V. Radiation therapy in primary carcinoma of the female urethra. II. An update on results. Cancer 1984;54:729.

54. Garden AS, Zagars GK, Delclos L. Primary carcinoma of the female urethra. Results of radiation therapy. Cancer 1993;71:3102.

55. Weghaupt K, Gerstner GJ, Kucera H. Radiation therapy for primary carcinoma of the female urethra: a survey over 25 years. Gynecol Oncol 1984;17:58.

56. Licht MR, Klein EA, Bukowski R, et al. Combination radiation and chemotherapy for the treatment of squamous cell carcinoma of the male and female urethra. J Urol 1918;153:1995.

57. Dalbagni G, Donat SM, Eschwege P, et al. Results of high dose rate brachytherapy, anterior pelvic exenteration and external beam radiotherapy for carcinoma of the female urethra. J Urol 2001;166:1759.

58. Ercole CE, Pow-Sang JM, Spiess PE. Update in the surgical principles and therapeutic outcomes of inguinal lymph node dissection for penile cancer. Urol Oncol 2013;31:505.

59. Milosevic MF, Warde PR, Banerjee D, et al. Urethral carcinoma in women: results of treatment with primary radiotherapy. Radiother Oncol 2000;56:29.

60. Grigsby PW. Carcinoma of the urethra in women. Int J Radiat Oncol Biol Phys 1998;41:535.

Management of Proximal Primary Urethral Cancer

Should Multidisciplinary Therapy Be the Gold Standard?

Leonard N. Zinman, MD, Alex J. Vanni, MD*

KEYWORDS

- Urethral carcinoma • Primary • Urethral cancer • Multimodal therapy • Surgery • Chemotherapy
- Radiotherapy

KEY POINTS

- Primary urethral cancer is rare, with proximal lesions accounting for 66% of diagnosed urethral tumors.
- Risk factors for survival include age, black race, tumor size, stage and grade, nodal involvement and metastasis, proximal location, histology, and the presence of concomitant bladder cancer.
- Patients with proximal urethral cancer who receive neoadjuvant multimodal therapy demonstrate improved survival compared with surgery with or without adjuvant chemotherapy.

INTRODUCTION

Primary urethral cancer (PUC) of the proximal urethra is an exceeding rare tumor, whose natural history is particularly aggressive. These tumors occur more commonly in men, and differ by location and histologic subtype. Patient symptoms often include urinary obstruction, irritative voiding symptoms, or hematuria. Risk factors include urethral strictures, chronic irritation, radiation treatment, human papilloma virus, and urethral diverticula (females). Most PUC are localized; however, 30% to 40% of patients present with regional lymph node metastasis. Although surgery and radiation treatment are options for early stage or distal urethral disease, advanced-stage and proximal PUC require multimodal treatment to optimize survival. However, controversy exists regarding the optimal multidisciplinary treatment strategy for male squamous cell carcinoma (SCC) of the urethra. Multi-institutional studies are critical to delineate the optimal treatment strategy in the future. This article examines this difficult disease, with a critical evaluation of the literature and an emphasis on the optimal treatment strategies for proximal PUC.

Epidemiology

PUC is exceeding rare, accounting for less than 1% of all malignancies.[1–3] The incidence of PUC increases with age, peaking in the greater than 75 year age group, and is more common in African Americans.[3] According to the Surveillance, Epidemiology, and End Results database, 4.3 per million and 1.5 per million men and women, respectively, in the United States develop PUC yearly.[3] This is slightly higher than the reported rates of PUC in Europe, where 1.6 per million men and 0.6 per million women develop PUC yearly.[2]

Etiology

The risk factors for developing PUC differ between men and women.[4–13] Risk factors for men include

Disclosure Statement: The authors have nothing to disclose.
Department of Urology, Lahey Hospital and Medical Center, Tufts University School of Medicine, 41 Mall Road, Burlington, MA 01805, USA
* Corresponding author.
E-mail address: alex.j.vanni@lahey.org

urethral stricture, chronic irritation from intermittent catheterization, prior radiation therapy, and sexually transmitted disease (human papillomavirus serotype 16). This is in contrast to women, whose risk factors for developing PUC include the following[14–17]: urethral diverticulum, chronic irritation and infection with human papillomavirus, and recurrent urinary tract infections.

Histology

The histologic subtypes of PUC reflect the gender and location of the primary tumor. In men, urothelial cancer is the most frequently seen histologic type, accounting for 47% to 73% of tumors, whereas SCC (12%–30%) and adenocarcinoma (5%–16%) account for the remaining cases.[2,3,18,19] Females have a slightly different incidence of tumor type. Although urothelial cancers are the most common, occurring in 45% of cases, adenocarcinoma is more prevalent than SCC, occurring in 29% and 19% of cases, respectively.[20]

Staging and Classification Systems

PUC is staged according to the TNM classification system, and is different depending on whether the tumor occurs in the prostatic urethra, or more distally[21] (**Table 1**). Although not directly measured by the TNM classification system, tumor location is an important factor that plays an integral role in PUC outcomes. PUC tumor locations are often referred to as occurring either proximally or distally. Although this is nonspecific nomenclature, its use has been propagated in the literature. Proximal PUC refer to tumors of the prostatic, membranous, and bulbar urethra, whereas distal tumors involve the penile and fossa navicularis urethra.

These anatomic considerations have treatment implications because of the varied lymphatic drainage of the urethra. The lymphatic drainage of the anterior urethra (bulbar, penile, and fossa navicularis urethra) is to the inguinal lymph nodes and subsequently pelvic lymph nodes, whereas the posterior urethra (prostatic and membranous urethra) drain into the pelvic lymph nodes. In women, the distal two-thirds drain into the superficial and deep inguinal lymph nodes, whereas the proximal third of the urethra drains into the pelvic lymph nodes.[22]

DIAGNOSIS
Presentation

Men may present with obstructive (41%–48%) or irritative urinary symptoms (20%), hematuria or

Table 1
TNM classification for urethral carcinoma

T: Primary Tumor	
Tx	Primary tumor cannot be assessed
Tis	Carcinoma in situ
T0	No evidence of primary tumor
T1	Tumor invades subepithelial connective tissue
T2	Tumor invades any of the following structures: corpus spongiosum, prostate, periurethral muscle
T3	Tumor invades any of the following structures: corpus cavernosum, invasion beyond prostatic capsule, anterior vaginal wall, bladder neck
T4	Tumor invades other adjacent organs
Primary Tumor in Prostatic Urethra	
Tx	Primary tumor cannot be assessed
Tis pu	Carcinoma in situ in the prostatic urethra
Tis pd	Carcinoma in situ in the prostatic ducts
T0	No evidence of primary tumor
T1	Tumor invades subepithelial connective tissue
T2	Tumor invades any of the following structures: corpus spongiosum, prostatic stroma, periurethral muscle
T3	Tumor invades any of the following structures: corpus cavernosum, beyond prostatic capsule, bladder neck
T4	Tumor invades other adjacent organs
N: Regional Lymph Nodes	
Nx	Regional lymph nodes cannot be assessed
N0	No regional lymph node metastases
N1	Metastasis in a single lymph node ≤2 cm in greatest dimension
N2	Metastasis in a single lymph node ≥3 cm in greatest dimension
M: Distant Metastasis	
Mx	Distant metastasis cannot be assessed
M0	No distant metastasis
M1	Distant metastasis

Abbreviations: M, metastasis; N, lymph nodes; Pd, prostatic ducts; Pu, prostatic urethra; T, tumor.

From Sobin LH, Gospodarowicz MK, Wittekind C, editors. TNM classification of malignant tumors. UICC International Union Against Cancer. 7th edition. Wiley-Blackwell; 2009.

urethral discharge (62%), pelvic pain (33%–45%), urethral stricture (76%), urethral/penile mass (48%–52%), urethrocutaneous fistula (10%), or abscess (5%).[23–26] More than 70% of women often report recurrent urinary tract infections, irritative voiding symptoms, spotting, or dyspareunia, whereas obstructive voiding (23%) and hematuria (20%) present less frequently.[27]

Physical Examination

A thorough physical examination that involves the external genitalia and rectal examination is mandatory in men, whereas women require a careful pelvic examination and palpation of the urethra. Both sexes should have bilateral inguinal evaluation to determine the presence of lymphadenopathy, and if present, whether the nodes are mobile. In cases of suspected PUC, an examination under anesthesia is important to properly stage the patient.

Tissue Diagnosis

Cystourethroscopy and biopsy are integral to confirm the diagnosis, establish the underlying histology and grade, determine the local extent of tumor, the precise location within the urethra, and whether a concomitant bladder tumor maybe present.[28] The biopsy technique required may be varied depending on the location of the PUC within the urethra. Although distal lesions may be simply excised for a tissue diagnosis, proximal tumors are more difficult. Cold-cup biopsy forceps can often be used to obtain a representative tumor sampling. In situations where this is technically demanding, we have found a 14-gauge Temno biopsy needle to be helpful. This is performed by activating the biopsy needle transurethrally (percutaneously). Urothelial tumors of the prostatic urethra are different, and are biopsied with the resectoscope loop, beginning at the bladder neck and ending proximal to the verumontanum to avoid any injury to the external sphincter and impair urinary continence.[29]

Imaging

Complete staging of patients with PUC requires imaging with either MRI or computed tomography of the chest, abdomen, and pelvis. MRI may be the preferred study because of its ability to accurately stage locoregional disease and distant metastases, and response to chemoradiation therapy.[30] A recent multi-institutional study confirmed these findings, demonstrating that 93% of clinically positive nodes on MRI were pathologically positive.[19] In cases of urothelial cancer, a computed tomography urogram should be performed to evaluate the entire urinary tract. The importance of accurate imaging cannot be underestimated, because 30% to 40% of all patients present with inguinal lymph node metastases, whereas up to 6% present with distant metastases.[18,20,22,24,27,31–33]

Prognosis

According to a Surveillance, Epidemiology, and End Results database analysis, the median 5- and 10-year overall survival of PUC is 46% and 29%, respectively, whereas the cancer-specific survival is 68% and 60%, respectively.[3] These rates are comparable with the findings of a European study that reported mean 1- and 5-year overall survival rates of 71% and 54%, respectively.[2] Despite the rarity of PUC, and the paucity of well-powered studies, several risk factors for decreased survival have been elucidated including the following[2,18–20,32]:

- Clinical stage, nodal involvement, grade, and metastases
- Proximal tumor location and size
- Tumor histology
- Treatment modality
- Age and black race
- Concomitant bladder tumor (patients with urothelial cancer)

However, the most important prognostic indicators as it relates to survival are clinical stage (presence of nodal metastasis) and location of the primary tumor (proximal vs distal).[18,19] Although treatment of lower stage tumors results in survival rates of 67% to 100%, the outcomes for patients with advanced disease is reported between 33% to 45%.[24,34,35] Similarly, survival rates for distal tumors is significantly better than for proximal PUC, with 60% to 72% of distal tumors and only 26% to 36% of proximal PUC demonstrating 5-year overall survival.[24,34,35] This disparity elucidates the very different behavior of these tumors, and ultimately the treatment required to maximize successful outcomes.

TREATMENT OF PROXIMAL PRIMARY URETHRAL CANCER
Urothelial Carcinoma of the Prostate

Several population-based studies have demonstrated that urothelial carcinoma of the prostatic urethra is the most common histologic type of cancer affecting the male urethra. Management of this disease entity is entirely different from the more aggressive SCC and adenocarcinoma of the proximal urethra, and is an extension of the management for urothelial cancer of the bladder. However, multimodal therapy remains the recommended treatment of clinical stage Ta or Tis prostatic urothelial carcinoma.[36,37]

Transurethral Resection and Bacillus Calmette-Guérin

In patients with Ta or Tis urothelial cancer, aggressive transurethral resection of the tumor followed by once weekly instillations of bacillus Calmette-Guérin (BCG) for 6 weeks is performed with durable results.[36,37] The complete response rate in the prostatic urethra and prostatic ducts has been shown in multiple small series to be 57% to 100% when transurethral resection is followed by intravesical BCG[36–41] (**Table 2**). This is significantly better than patients who only receive monotherapy BCG (65% complete response rate).[40] However, up to 55% of patients who experienced a complete response later developed recurrence in either the urethra or bladder. In these limited studies, 28% to 30% of patients ultimately required cystoprostatectomy and urinary diversion for recurrent or progressive disease.[36,37] In this highly select group, at a median follow-up of 7.5 years, disease-specific survival was 89% with this multimodal approach.[36,37,40]

Radical Cystoprostatectomy

In addition to the 28% to 30% of patients with superficial prostatic urothelial cancer who will ultimately require radical cystoprostatectomy, patients with extensive prostatic ductal involvement or stromal invasion should be offered radical cystoprostatectomy with extended pelvic lymphadenectomy and urinary diversion.[41–43] An extended pelvic lymphadenectomy in these patients should be considered, because 50% of patients in one study demonstrated positive lymph nodes situated above the iliac bifurcation.[43]

MULTIMODAL THERAPY VERSUS MONOTHERAPY FOR PROXIMAL URETHRAL CANCER

Because of the paucity of robust data evaluating patients with proximal PUC, definitive conclusions about the best therapy remain elusive. Treatment algorithms, chemotherapy regimens, surgical templates, and follow-up times vary dramatically within the published literature, making comparisons of different treatment modalities difficult. Despite the lack of prospective, multicenter data, the preponderance of evidence supports the use of multimodal therapy for proximal PUC.

Monotherapy

Treatment of male and female urethral cancer has historically been with surgical excision. However, the outcomes of surgical therapy for male proximal PUC have been dismal because of the difficulty achieving local control.[44] Local recurrence rates are high, ranging from 50% to 57% in two small retrospective studies.[24,34] Even aggressive surgical resection with pelvic exenteration with or without pelvic lymph node dissection resulted in a 63% local recurrence rate.[33,34,45,46] Likewise, survival rates for surgical monotherapy for proximal PUC have been reported between 0% and 38%.[24,33,34,45–47]

Radiation monotherapy has similarly dismal results, with a 0% to 25% 5-year survival for penile urethral tumors.[24,46,48] Although there is a paucity of data for proximal PUC treated with radiation monotherapy, extrapolation of the poor performance for distal PUC precludes recommendation for this method of treatment.

Although surgical monotherapy with resection or complete urethrectomy for distal urethral cancers in women provides reasonable recurrence-free survival, women with advanced or proximal tumors have poor outcomes.[28] Pelvic exenteration in women with advanced tumors demonstrated only an 11% to 42% overall 5-year survival rate.[27,49–52] Similarly, radiation monotherapy in women with distal urethral cancer has demonstrated a 64% local control rate and a 49% 7-year cancer-specific survival.[53] However, in several small studies, the overall 5-year survival rate of radiation monotherapy continues to be poor (0%–50%).[54–56]

Table 2
Outcomes for prostatic urothelial carcinoma: transurethral resection with BCG

Study	Patients	Follow-up (mo)	Prostate Response (%)	Required Cystectomy (%)	Overall Survival (%)
Palou Redorta et al,[36] 2006	11	27	82	30	91
Taylor et al,[37] 2007	28	90	64.3	28	89
Gofrit et al,[40] 2009	20	52.5	90	25	66
Hillyard et al,[41] 1988	8	22.3	75	25	—

Multimodal Therapy

Despite the lack of large, multi-institutional trials, there is a preponderance of data from multiple single institution series demonstrating superior recurrence-free and survival data for patients treated with multimodal therapy (**Table 3**). The critical questions remaining are which combinations and timing of chemotherapy, radiation therapy, and surgery will result in the best overall results for patients with proximal PUC.

Surgery and Adjuvant Radiotherapy

Although the data for surgery or radiation monotherapy are poor, combining adjuvant radiation following pelvic exenteration with or without lymphadenectomy improves local control. Men with proximal PUC who underwent pelvic exenteration with or without lymphadenectomy had a local recurrence rate of 63%. In this group of studies, the local recurrence rate dropped to 24% when men had a pelvic exenteration (with en bloc resection of the pubis) with or without lymphadenectomy and adjuvant radiation therapy.[34,46,57,58] Although, radiation therapy may minimize local recurrence, these studies are confounded by the change in surgical technique. The more extensive resection in the latter group of patients may have also contributed to the improved local control.

The largest group of patients with proximal PUC who underwent extensive surgical resection with either cystoprostatectomy or penectomy with adjuvant radiation with or without chemotherapy demonstrated a 5-year overall survival rate of only 36%, and a disease-free rate of 15%.[35]

Lastly, adjuvant radiation has the potential for significant side effects and complications including urethral stricture, tissue necrosis, fistula, and edema.[24,46,48]

Radiation Therapy and Surgery

Dalbagni and colleagues[24] published the largest series of male patients with urethral cancer, which included 46 men. Forty men had surgery alone, and six men had radiation therapy followed by salvage surgery. A total of 48% of patients had T3 or T4 disease and 22% presented with positive lymph nodes. The overall and disease-specific survival rates at 5 years were 42% and 50%, respectively. Because only six patients had this form of multimodal therapy, no definitive conclusions are inferred from this work.

Perioperative Chemotherapy

In the last two decades, platinum-based perioperative chemotherapy regimens for advanced PUC have become the mainstay of treatment at most academic centers. Unfortunately, there is not a uniform standard of treatment across centers, making data interpretation difficult.

Dayyani and colleagues[59] published a study of 44 patients (16 men, 28 women), 21 of whom received platinum-based preoperative chemotherapy followed by surgery. A total of 98% of patients had T3 or T4 disease and 59% had positive lymph nodes. Unfortunately, the PUC were not classified according to location. Preoperative chemotherapy was cisplatin, gemcitabine, and ifosfomide for SCC; methotrexate, vinblastine, doxorubicin, and cisplatin for urothelial tumors; and 5-fluorouracil, gemcitabine, and cisplatin for adenocarcinoma. This approach demonstrated a 72% response rate, and median overall survival of 32 months. However, overall survival was 46 months in patients who underwent surgery. There was not adequate follow-up to calculate a 5-year survival.

A recent multi-institutional study of 26 patients with cT3 and/or node-positive disease demonstrated improved relapse-free and overall survival in the group who had either neoadjuvant chemotherapy or neoadjuvant radiotherapy compared with those who had surgery alone or surgery and adjuvant chemotherapy.[5] Although, only eight total patients received either neoadjuvant chemotherapy or chemoradiotherapy, all eight patients were alive at 5 years. In addition to improved relapse-free and overall survival, the same patients receiving neoadjuvant chemoradiotherapy had a lower rate of cystectomy compared with patients who received adjuvant chemotherapy despite similar rates of pathologically advanced disease.[5] This finding illustrates the potential positive effect of tumor downstaging, thereby improving the subsequent surgical resection. Additionally, of the 39 total patients in the study who had perioperative chemotherapy (including distal tumors), proximal tumor location correlated with a worse 3-year relapse-free and overall survival.[5]

In both of these studies, patients who had preoperative cisplatin-based chemotherapy had improved overall survival compared with patients treated with chemotherapy alone.[5,19,59] Although these studies have small patient numbers, they elucidate the important concept of neoadjuvant cisplatin-based chemoradiotherapy before surgery as the preferred therapeutic approach for advanced PUC.

Chemoradiotherapy and Salvage Surgery

Patients who desire organ preservation have limited options for treatment. Preoperative local

Table 3
Outcomes of multimodal therapy for advanced or proximal urethral cancer

Study	Thyavihally et al,[35] 2006	Dalbagni et al,[24] 1999	Dayyani et al,[59] 2013	Kent et al,[23] 2015	Gakis et al,[5] 2015
Patients	36 Proximal: 17	40 Proximal: 26	44 (98% T3/T4 or N+)	26 (88% T3/T4 or N+)	Proximal: 26
Surgery alone	4	40	3	—	10
Chemotherapy + surgery	3	—	24	—	5
Chemoradiation + surgery	—	—	—	—	3
Surgery + radiation	12	—	—	—	—
Radiation + surgery	—	6	—	—	—
Surgery + chemotherapy	6	—	1	—	8
Chemotherapy + radiation	—	—	—	26	—
Chemotherapy	—	—	15	—	—
Overall survival	Proximal 5 y: 36% Total 5 y: 49%	Proximal 5 y: 26% Total 5 y: 42%	Median 31.7 mo	5 y: 52%	3 y: 61% 100% in chemoradiation + surgery group (n = 8)
Disease-free survival	Proximal 5 y: 15% Total 5 y: 23%	—	—	5 y: 43%	—
Local recurrence-free survival (%)	—	Total 5 y: 51%	—	—	—
Metastasis-free survival (%)	—	Total 5 y: 56%	—	—	—

Abbreviations: chemoradiation, chemotherapy and radiation therapy; N+, lymph node positive.

radiotherapy with concurrent radiosensitizing chemotherapy is an alternative to surgery in locally advanced SCC of the urethra.[23,60–62] The preoperative radiation field includes the inguinal and pelvic lymph node regions and genitalia. A total of 45 to 55 Gy is delivered with a 12- to 15-Gy boost to the primary tumor. Concurrent chemotherapy with a combination of 5-fluorouracil (Days 1–4 and 29) and mitomycin-C (Days 1 and 29) is delivered. A recent study of 26 patients underwent the chemoradiotherapy protocol, with 88% of patients having cT3 $\pm$ node-positive disease. The 5-year overall and disease-specific survival rates were 52% and 68%, respectively.[23] A total of 79% of patients demonstrated a complete response, with 42% of these patients having a delayed recurrence at a median of 12.5 months. Of the 21% of patients who did not respond to treatment and had salvage surgery, all died of their disease.[23] It should be noted that the median overall survival of this cohort was 35.5 months, which is similar to the overall survival in the largest series of neoadjuvant chemotherapy and surgery by Dayyani and colleagues (31.7 months).[23,59] All of the patients developed some degree of posttreatment urethral stricture, with 53% of patients requiring complex urethral reconstruction.

Patients considering this genital-sparing technique need to be carefully counseled about the risk of disease recurrence and overall disease-specific mortality and balance this with the opportunity of genital preservation.

SUMMARY

There are several caveats that are important as it pertains to chemoradiation therapy. Although this multimodal therapy seems to have equivalent oncologic outcomes compared with neoadjuvant chemotherapy and surgery, these data pertain to SCC of the urethra only. Other forms of PUC, such as urothelial cancer and adenocarcinoma, are not candidates for this type of multimodal therapy, and should be offered other forms of treatment. For patients with proximal SCC of the urethra, chemoradiation seems to offer comparable oncologic control while potentially preserving the patent's genitals.

Additionally, further study is needed to determine whether all patients should receive consolidation surgery following chemoradiation. The data presented by Kent and colleagues[23] demonstrated a delayed 42% recurrence rate (median, 12.5 months) in complete responders. Although the overall survival between chemoradiation and neoadjuvant chemotherapy and surgery seem comparable for SCC, consolidation surgery may

further improve the survival rates for patients undergoing chemoradiation. Further study should focus on consolidation surgery in this particular treatment modality.

Multidisciplinary therapy, in the form of either neoadjuvant chemotherapy and surgery or chemoradiotherapy and salvage surgery, has clearly improved the local recurrence rates and overall survival of proximal PUC. For these reasons, we believe multidisciplinary therapy is the gold standard treatment of proximal PUC. However, there continues to be many unanswered questions regarding the optimal multimodal therapy for this devastating disease, which can only be answered with prospective multi-institutional studies.

REFERENCES

1. Gatta G, van der Zwan JM, Casali PG, et al. Rare cancers are not so rare: the rare cancer burden in Europe. Eur J Cancer 2011;47(17):2493–511.
2. Visser O, Adolfsson J, Rossi S, et al. Incidence and survival of rare urogenital cancers in Europe. Eur J Cancer 2012;48(4):456–64.
3. Swartz MA, Porter MP, Lin DW, et al. Incidence of primary urethral carcinoma in the United States. Urology 2006;68(6):1164–8.
4. Medina Perez M, Valero Puerta J, Sanchez Gonzalez M, et al. Squamous carcinoma of the male urethra, its presentation as a scrotal abscess. Arch Esp Urol 1999;52(7):792–4 [in Spanish].
5. Gakis G, Morgan TM, Daneshmand S, et al. Impact of perioperative chemotherapy on survival in patients with advanced primary urethral cancer: results of the international collaboration on primary urethral carcinoma. Ann Oncol 2015;26(8):1754–9.
6. Van de Voorde W, Meertens B, Baert L, et al. Urethral squamous cell carcinoma associated with urethral stricture and urethroplasty. Eur J Surg Oncol 1994; 20(4):478–83.
7. Colapinto V, Evans DH. Primary carcinoma of the male urethra developing after urethroplasty for stricture. J Urol 1977;118(4):581–4.
8. Mohanty NK, Jolly BB, Saxena S, et al. Squamous cell carcinoma of perineal urethrostomy. Urol Int 1995;55(2):118–9.
9. Sawczuk I, Acosta R, Grant D, et al. Post urethroplasty squamous cell carcinoma. N Y State J Med 1986;86(5):261–3.
10. Mohan H, Bal A, Punia RP, et al. Squamous cell carcinoma of the prostate. Int J Urol 2003;10(2):114–6.
11. Arva NC, Das K. Diagnostic dilemmas of squamous differentiation in prostate carcinoma case report and review of the literature. Diagn Pathol 2011;6:46.
12. Cupp MR, Malek RS, Goellner JR, et al. Detection of human papillomavirus DNA in primary squamous

cell carcinoma of the male urethra. Urology 1996; 48(4):551–5.

13. Wiener JS, Liu ET, Walther PJ. Oncogenic human papillomavirus type 16 is associated with squamous cell cancer of the male urethra. Cancer Res 1992; 52(18):5018–23.

14. Ahmed K, Dasgupta R, Vats A, et al. Urethral diverticular carcinoma: an overview of current trends in diagnosis and management. Int Urol Nephrol 2010; 42(2):331–41.

15. Chung DE, Purohit RS, Girshman J, et al. Urethral diverticula in women: discrepancies between magnetic resonance imaging and surgical findings. J Urol 2010;183(6):2265–9.

16. Thomas AA, Rackley RR, Lee U, et al. Urethral diverticula in 90 female patients: a study with emphasis on neoplastic alterations. J Urol 2008; 180(6):2463–7.

17. Libby B, Chao D, Schneider BF. Non-surgical treatment of primary female urethral cancer. Rare Tumors 2010;2(3):e55.

18. Rabbani F. Prognostic factors in male urethral cancer. Cancer 2011;117(11):2426–34.

19. Gakis G, Morgan TM, Efstathiou JA, et al. Prognostic factors and outcomes in primary urethral cancer: results from the international collaboration on primary urethral carcinoma. World J Urol 2016;34(1):97–103.

20. Derksen JW, Visser O, de la Riviere GB, et al. Primary urethral carcinoma in females: an epidemiologic study on demographical factors, histological types, tumour stage and survival. World J Urol 2013;31(1):147–53.

21. Sorbin LH, Gospodarowicz MK, Wittekind C, editors. TNM classification of malignant tumors. UICC International Union Against Cancer. 7th edition. Chichester (United Kingdom): Wiley-Blackwell; 2009.

22. Carroll PR, Dixon CM. Surgical anatomy of the male and female urethra. Urol Clin North Am 1992;19(2): 339–46.

23. Kent M, Zinman L, Girshovich L, et al. Combined chemoradiation as primary treatment for invasive male urethral cancer. J Urol 2015;193(2):532–7.

24. Dalbagni G, Zhang ZF, Lacombe L, et al. Male urethral carcinoma: analysis of treatment outcome. Urology 1999;53(6):1126–32.

25. Gheiler EL, Tefilli MV, Tiguert R, et al. Management of primary urethral cancer. Urology 1998;52(3):487–93.

26. Golijanin D, Yossepowitch O, Beck SD, et al. Carcinoma in a bladder diverticulum: presentation and treatment outcome. J Urol 2003;170(5):1761–4.

27. Dalbagni G, Zhang ZF, Lacombe L, et al. Female urethral carcinoma: an analysis of treatment outcome and a plea for a standardized management strategy. Br J Urol 1998;82(6):835–41.

28. Gakis G, Witjes JA, Comperat E, et al. EAU guidelines on primary urethral carcinoma. Eur Urol 2013; 64(5):823–30.

29. Donat SM, Wei DC, McGuire MS, et al. The efficacy of transurethral biopsy for predicting the long-term clinical impact of prostatic invasive bladder cancer. J Urol 2001;165(5):1580–4.

30. Gourtsoyianni S, Hudolin T, Sala E, et al. MRI at the completion of chemoradiotherapy can accurately evaluate the extent of disease in women with advanced urethral carcinoma undergoing anterior pelvic exenteration. Clin Radiol 2011;66(11):1072–8.

31. Anderson KA, McAninch JW. Primary squamous cell carcinoma of anterior male urethra. Urology 1984; 23(2):134–40.

32. Champ CE, Hegarty SE, Shen X, et al. Prognostic factors and outcomes after definitive treatment of female urethral cancer: a population-based analysis. Urology 2012;80(2):374–81.

33. Ray B, Canto AR, Whitmore WF Jr. Experience with primary carcinoma of the male urethra. J Urol 1977;117(5):591–4.

34. Dinney CP, Johnson DE, Swanson DA, et al. Therapy and prognosis for male anterior urethral carcinoma: an update. Urology 1994;43(4):506–14.

35. Thyavihally YB, Tongaonkar HB, Srivastava SK, et al. Clinical outcome of 36 male patients with primary urethral carcinoma: a single center experience. Int J Urol 2006;13(6):716–20.

36. Palou Redorta J, Schatteman P, Huguet Perez J, et al. Intravesical instillations with bacillus Calmette-Guerin for the treatment of carcinoma in situ involving prostatic ducts. Eur Urol 2006;49(5): 834–8 [discussion: 838].

37. Taylor JH, Davis J, Schellhammer P. Long-term follow-up of intravesical bacillus Calmette-Guerin treatment for superficial transitional-cell carcinoma of the bladder involving the prostatic urethra. Clin Genitourin Cancer 2007;5(6):386–9.

38. Palou J, Baniel J, Klotz L, et al. Urothelial carcinoma of the prostate. Urology 2007;69(1 Suppl):50–61.

39. Njinou Ngninkeu B, Lorge F, Moulin P, et al. Transitional cell carcinoma involving the prostate: a clinicopathological retrospective study of 76 cases. J Urol 2003;169(1):149–52.

40. Gofrit ON, Pode D, Pizov G, et al. Prostatic urothelial carcinoma: is transurethral prostatectomy necessary before bacillus Calmette-Guerin immunotherapy? BJU Int 2009;103(7):905–8.

41. Hillyard RW Jr, Ladaga L, Schellhammer PF. Superficial transitional cell carcinoma of the bladder associated with mucosal involvement of the prostatic urethra: results of treatment with intravesical bacillus Calmette-Guerin. J Urol 1988;139(2):290–3.

42. Solsona E, Iborra I, Ricos JV, et al. The prostate involvement as prognostic factor in patients with superficial bladder tumors. J Urol 1995;154(5):1710–3.

43. Vazina A, Dugi D, Shariat SF, et al. Stage specific lymph node metastasis mapping in radical cystectomy specimens. J Urol 2004;171(5):1830–4.

44. Smith Y, Hadway P, Ahmed S, et al. Penile-preserving surgery for male distal urethral carcinoma. BJU Int 2007;100(1):82–7.

45. Farrer JH, Lupu AN. Carcinoma of deep male urethra. Urology 1984;24(6):527–31.

46. Bracken RB, Henry R, Ordonez N. Primary carcinoma of the male urethra. South Med J 1980;73(8): 1003–5.

47. Mandler JI, Pool TL. Primary carcinoma of the male urethra. J Urol 1966;96(1):67–72.

48. Kaplan GW, Bulkey GJ, Grayhack JT. Carcinoma of the male urethra. J Urol 1967;98(3):365–71.

49. Grabstald H. Proceedings: tumors of the urethra in men and women. Cancer 1973;32(5):1236–55.

50. Srinivas V, Khan SA. Female urethral cancer: an overview. Int Urol Nephrol 1987;19(4):423–7.

51. Desai S, Libertino JA, Zinman L. Primary carcinoma of the female urethra. J Urol 1973;110(6):693–5.

52. Peterson DT, Dockerty MB, Utz DC, et al. The peril of primary carcinoma of the urethra in women. J Urol 1973;110(1):72–5.

53. Garden AS, Zagars GK, Delclos L. Primary carcinoma of the female urethra. Results of radiation therapy. Cancer 1993;71(10):3102–8.

54. Weghaupt K, Gerstner GJ, Kucera H. Radiation therapy for primary carcinoma of the female urethra: a survey over 25 years. Gynecol Oncol 1984;17(1):58–63.

55. Chu AM. Female urethral carcinoma. Radiology 1973;107(3):627–30.

56. Hahn P, Krepart G, Malaker K. Carcinoma of female urethra. Manitoba experience: 1958-1987. Urology 1991;37(2):106–9.

57. Klein FA, Whitmore WF Jr, Herr HW, et al. Inferior pubic rami resection with en bloc radical excision for invasive proximal urethral carcinoma. Cancer 1983; 51(7):1238–42.

58. Shuttleworth KE, Lloyd-Davies RW. Radical resection for tumours involving the posterior urethra. Br J Urol 1969;41(6):739–43.

59. Dayyani F, Pettaway CA, Kamat AM, et al. Retrospective analysis of survival outcomes and the role of cisplatin-based chemotherapy in patients with urethral carcinomas referred to medical oncologists. Urol Oncol 2013;31(7): 1171–7.

60. Cohen MS, Triaca V, Billmeyer B, et al. Coordinated chemoradiation therapy with genital preservation for the treatment of primary invasive carcinoma of the male urethra. J Urol 2008;179(2):536–41 [discussion: 541].

61. Itoh J, Mitsuzuka K, Kimura S, et al. Docetaxel, cisplatin and 5-fluorouracil chemotherapy with concurrent radiation for unresectable advanced urethral carcinoma. Int J Urol 2014;21(4):422–4.

62. Gakis G. Editorial Comment to docetaxel, cisplatin and 5-fluorouracil chemotherapy with concurrent radiation for unresectable advanced urethral carcinoma. Int J Urol 2014;21(4):424–5.

Management of Urethral Recurrences
Urothelial and Nonurothelial

Kamran Zargar-Shoshtari, MBChB, MD, FRACS[a], Wade J. Sexton, MD[b], Michael A. Poch, MD[b],*

KEYWORDS

• Urethra • Urothelial carcinoma • Squamous cell carcinoma • Recurrence • Organ preservation
• Therapy

KEY POINTS

- Urethral carcinoma is a rare disease and may present as primary cancer or be associated with disease of the bladder at the time of cystectomy.
- There are relatively more data on management of urethral recurrence following cystectomy for urothelial carcinoma of the bladder.
- Urethral metachronous relapses have been managed with both urethra preserving as well as urethrectomy.
- There are minimal data on management of relapse following primary urethral carcinoma. The management options are similar to those seen with primary urethral cancer.
- Multimodal therapies with chemotherapy and radiation should be considered in more advanced disease.

INTRODUCTION

Urethral carcinoma can be encountered in the settings of primary urethral cancer, synchronous presentation with other genitourinary (GU) malignancies, relapse following primary urethral cancer, or metachronous recurrence after treatment of other GU malignancies. Regardless of clinical situation and presentation, there are comparatively few data on treatment options for primary and recurrent urethral cancer. There are no prospective studies in the management of urethral carcinoma, and the current information is largely based on retrospective experience, often from single institutions.[1]

This article will review some of the reported therapeutic strategies in the management of recurrent urethral carcinoma. It describes treatment options in recurrences encountered following cystectomy as well as relapse following treatment for primary urethral cancer.

URETHRAL RECURRENCE AFTER CYSTECTOMY

Prophylactic urethrectomy at the time of radical cystectomy for urothelial carcinoma is often performed in patients who are considered to be at high risk for urethral recurrence. Certain contemporary indications for prophylactic urethrectomy in men include cystectomy for nonmuscle invasive bladder cancer (NMIBC), history of recurrent NMIBC, involvement of the prostatic urethra by urothelial cancer, or microscopic involvement of the urethra based on positive intraoperative urethral frozen sections.[2] In female patients, cancer at the bladder neck or cancer involving the anterior

Disclosures: None.
[a] Division of Urology, Department of Surgery, University of Auckland, Auckland, New Zealand; [b] Department of Genitourinary Oncology, Moffitt Cancer Center, 12902 Magnolia Drive, Tampa, FL 33612, USA
* Corresponding author.
E-mail address: michael.poch@moffitt.org

Urol Clin N Am 43 (2016) 515–521
http://dx.doi.org/10.1016/j.ucl.2016.06.012

vaginal wall is associated with an increased risk of urethral recurrence.[3,4]

It is reported that following radical cystectomy, new urethral tumors occur in 1.5% to 6% of men and 6% to 11% of women. Some have suggested that the incidence of urothelial recurrence in the female urethra may be lower, possibly related to prominence of squamous mucosa in the female urethra.[5] Furthermore, the incidence of urethral recurrence is reportedly also lower in both men and women treated with neobladder reconstruction (1%–4%).[6–8] Most urethral recurrences occur within 24 months after surgery, with reported median time to relapse of 8 to 28 months.[9] In a report that included 7 patients with neobladder substitution who had initial negative intraoperative frozen sections but positive urethral margins at final pathology, only 1 patient subsequently developed recurrence in the urethra.[1] Similarly, of 136 patients with moderate-to-severe atypia or positive urethral margins, only 5 patients (3.7%) subsequently developed urethral recurrence.[10]

Lower incidence of urethral recurrence in patients with neobladders may to some extent relate to selection bias, with lower-risk patients or those with negative bladder neck or prostatic urethral margins being selected for neobladder diversion. However, some authors have suggested that even after controlling for potential risk factors such as tumor grade and multifocality, carcinoma in situ, and pathologic stage, as well as prostatic involvement, patients with neobladder diversions may still have lower adjusted rates for urethral recurrence compared with cutaneous diversions.[11,12] Others have suggested urine remaining in contact with the urothelium may be protective or that juxtaposition of the ilium to the urethra may provide a degree of protection, although none of these purposed mechanisms has been proven.[6]

The detection and diagnosis of urethral recurrence following radical cystectomy can be secondary to symptomatic presentation or detection through routine surveillance with urethral wash cytology or endoscopic examination.

One reported technique for performing a urethral wash involves the insertion of a minimally lubricated 14 French (Fr) catheter into the proximal penile urethra, followed by irrigation of 100 mL of normal saline solution and collection of all extruded solution at the level of the urethral meatus. The catheter should be withdrawn gradually and removed while flushing continues (**Fig. 1**).[13]

The value of routine surveillance, however, is questioned by some, as there is evidence that positive urethral wash cytology may not improve survival. In several case series, patients experienced similar survival rates, regardless of whether they received treatment following diagnosis based on symptoms (bleeding, urethral discharge, pain, or palpable mass) or based primarily on positive urethral cytology.[14–16] It has also been suggested that while asymptomatic patients diagnosed by cytology might have a higher chance of harboring noninvasive disease, overall survival may not be significantly better than survival in symptomatic patients with invasive (pT1-pT4) cancer.[17] On the contrary, others have demonstrated that noninvasive recurrences have a favorable prognosis when detected early,[18] and there is evidence that patients who present with symptomatic urethral

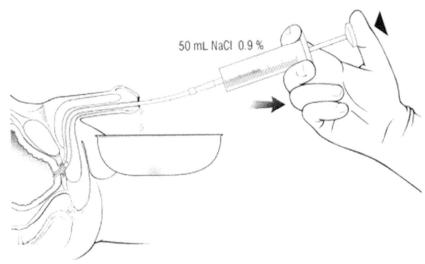

50 mL NaCl 0.9 %

Fig. 1. Technique for performing a urethral wash for cytology. (*From* Varol C, Thalmann GN, Burkhard FC, et al. Treatment of urethral recurrence following radical cystectomy and ileal bladder substitution. J Urol 2004;172(3):937–42; with permission.)

recurrences have significantly worse survival than those who present asymptomatically, most likely related to more advanced or potentially metastatic disease at presentation.[2] An additional advantage of urethra wash cytology may be diagnosis at an earlier stage, permitting urethral preservation.[19]

Management of urethral recurrence is dictated by disease stage, grade and location, patient comorbidities, the type of diversion, as well as the presence or absence of systemic disease.

Urethral preserving approaches, both with orthotopic and cutaneous diversions, have been described. In a series of 15 urethral recurrences in patients with previous cystectomy and orthotopic neobladder reconstruction, 10 patients were treated with intraurethral bacillus Calmette-Guérin (BCG). In this series, all but one of the patients were diagnosed through surveillance with urethral wash cytology.[13]

The technique of intraurethral BCG administration involved modification of an existing 14 Fr Foley catheter where the catheter just distal to the Foley balloon was ligated to occlude the drainage holes. Instead, 5 new irrigation openings were cut in the lumen of the catheter over a 2 to 3 cm length, starting approximately 0.5 cm proximal to the balloon. This nonlubricated catheter was subsequently inserted into the bladder and the balloon inflated to 10 mLs of fluid. Thereafter 100 mL of standard concentration of BCG was infused at 20 cm of water pressure over 75 minutes, with the patient changing position during urethral irrigation. Once the irrigation was completed, the catheter was removed, and another 25 mLs of standard concentration BCG was instilled into the urethra and penile clamp placed to facilitate topical contact of the BCG with the urethra for an additional 25 minutes. This was repeated again with another 25 mLs of BCG solution (**Fig. 2**). This treatment approach was utilized for 6 weeks total.

No systemic adverse effects were reported in patients treated with this technique. Five of 6 men with new urethral carcinoma in situ (CIS) responded to intraurethral BCG therapy, whereas none of the 4 patients with papillary disease responded to the treatment. Subsequently, patients with CIS who responded to BCG had significantly longer survival (85 months compared with 26 months).[13] Investigators from a subsequent publication reported a 92% response rate using this technique in 13 patients with recurrence of urethral CIS.[19]

Several small series have described transurethral resection (TUR) and fulguration without BCG therapy in patients with clinical Ta and clinical T1 tumor recurrences, with reported satisfactory local response rates.[20–22] However, in another report of 4 patients treated with TUR and no topical therapy, 3 patients eventually required urethrectomy.[20] Overall, topical ablative therapies should only be considered in selected cases, where tumors or tumor volumes are considered small, adequately accessible, and with a good chance for complete excision or destruction.

Distal urethrectomy with perineal urethrostomy has also been described in patients with urethral recurrence after neobladder diversion. In a series of five such cases, 2 patients subsequently required total urethrectomy. Nevertheless, a subtotal urethrectomy remains an option in selected cases.[16]

In situations where urethral preservation is not feasible, urethrectomy should be considered. In men with orthotopic neobladder substitutions, conversion to an ileal conduit may be necessary. Long-term outcomes in these patients will depend on local stage and likelihood of metastatic progression. In a relatively large series, 49 patients with recurrent urethral tumors following cystectomy were treated with urethrectomy. Of these patients, 57% eventually died of disease. At a median follow-up of

A　　　　　　　　　　　　**B**

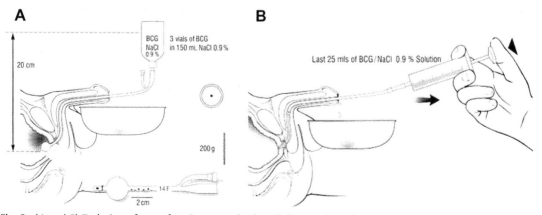

Fig. 2. (*A* and *B*) Technique for performing a urethral wash for cytology. (*From* Varol C, Thalmann GN, Burkhard FC, et al. Treatment of urethral recurrence following radical cystectomy and ileal bladder substitution. J Urol 2004;172(3):937–42; with permission.)

38 months, disease-specific survival rates were 85%, 65%, and 55% at 2, 3, and 5 years, respectively. The authors demonstrated that symptomatic presentations, and earlier recurrences were associated with worse survival outcomes.[10]

Akkad and colleagues described 4 urethral recurrences following radical cystectomy in female patients. Two of the patients had orthotopic neobladders, and 2 patients had ileal conduit diversions. All were treated with urethrectomy, with conversion of neobladders to ileal conduits. Patients without metastatic disease had good long-term outcomes.[23]

URETHRAL RECURRENCE FOLLOWING NONUROTHELIAL CARCINOMA

The rate of urethral recurrence may be lower in patients with pure squamous cell carcinoma compared with urothelial carcinoma. In a multi-institutional study involving female patients treated with neobladder substitutions, only one of 126 patients with pure SCC developed urethral recurrence compared with 6 of 151 patents with nonsquamous urothelial cancers. The authors suggested that higher urethral relapse, despite similar pelvic and systemic relapse, may be related to changes in tumor biology and the cancer field defect of the urothelium described in patients with urothelial carcinoma.[1]

RECURRENCE FOLLOWING TREATMENT OF PRIMARY URETHRAL CARCINOMA

The rate of local recurrence in patients previously treated by urethral preservation varies, depending on the initial disease stage and the therapeutic regimen(s) administered. There are no data describing specific therapeutic options in this patient group, and management is mainly based on the experiences derived from treatment of primary urethral cancers.

In men with cancer recurrences involving the distal penile urethra, organ-preserving strategies may still be feasible, and the options potentially include transurethral resection, local excision, or distal urethrectomy and perineal urethrostomy. These may provide adequate treatment in selected patients with low-grade, noninvasive recurrences.[24] More locally advanced disease (T2 or higher) located in the distal urethra and penis may be treated with partial penectomy as long as negative surgical margins can be achieved. However, total urethrectomy may be required in patients with carcinoma extending to the more proximal urethra where tumor-free margins may not be possible. In men with anterior urethral pT1-3 N0-2 disease following partial penectomy, local recurrence was not observed as long as surgical resection margins were negative, even if the tumor-free margin was less than 5 mm.[25] The management of penile corporal bodies at the time of surgery will depend on the local extent of the urethral disease. In situations where the tumor is confined to the urethra and the corpus spongiosum, and there is no involvement of the corpora cavernosa, excision of the urethra and corpus spongiosum alone may provide adequate oncological control, allowing for preservation of all or parts of the corpora cavernosa and penis.[26,27]

Recurrences in the bulbar urethra may be more complicated, and require more careful assessment and treatment planning. In patients who present with low-volume, noninvasive disease, transurethral resection or partial excision of the urethra with primary anastomosis has been described, although these are mainly in the primary setting. Overall, suitable candidates for local therapies are not encountered commonly, as most men with bulbar urethral carcinoma present in a delayed fashion with advanced disease. In a majority of men presenting with relapse at the bulbar urethra, radical cystoprostatectomy with total urethrectomy or even radical penectomy penectomy might be required along with adequate lymph node resection for both staging and therapeutic purposes.[28]

TREATMENT OPTIONS IN FEMALES WITH RECURRENT URETHRAL CARCINOMA

In the absence of bulky relapse, the distal third of the female urethra may be excised without significant impact on urinary continence. Therefore, circumferential excision of the urethra and the anterior vaginal wall may be an option in female patients who present with small distal lesions, near the meatus. If partial excision is being considered, frozen section sampling must be performed to ensure complete excision with negative surgical margins. Partial urethrectomy in female patients is associated with incontinence in approximately 40% of cases.[29]

Attempts to preserve the urethra in the setting of more advanced disease recurrence (T2-3), may result in suboptimal oncological control, with a relatively high risk for local recurrence approaching 20%, even in patients treated for T2 disease in the primary setting. Overall, urethral preservation when there is recurrent, locally advanced disease is challenging.[29] However, clinical data in patients with primary disease suggest that even in presence of more advanced urethral tumor, bladder preservation could still be an option with acceptable rates of local control. These patients should be treated initially with primary radical urethrectomy, including excision of the entire periurethral tissue from the bulbocavernosus muscles extending proximally to the pubic symphysis and the bladder neck. After urethral excision, the bladder neck should be closed, and a catheterizable proximal diversion such as an appendicovesicostomy or an ileovesicostomy could be considered. In the presence of recurrent disease, the feasibility of the latter treatment strategies will depend of the primary treatment administered, the local impact of the primary treatment, as well as the patient's overall health status.[29–31] More extensive disease necessitates cystectomy with wide excision of the urethra, followed by urinary diversion.[29]

MULTIMODAL THERAPY: THE ROLE OF RADIATION AND CHEMOTHERAPY

There are recent data demonstrating that contemporary platinum-based chemotherapy regimens are beneficial in the management of primary urethral cancers. Combination chemotherapy and radiation might also be applicable in patients with recurrent urethral tumors. In a retrospective study of 44 patients with primary urethral carcinoma (39% squamous cell, 30% adenocarcinoma, 19% urothelial, 18% mixed/other; 98% T3-T4, 43% N+, and 16% M+), a 72% pathologic response rate to neoadjuvant chemotherapy was observed. Patients who underwent surgery after chemotherapy had significantly improved overall survival compared with those who were managed with chemotherapy alone.[32]

The combination of chemosensitizing 5-fluorouracil or mitomycin-C concurrent with 25 fractions (45–55 Gy) of radiation has also been reported in 25 men with squamous cell carcinoma (88% cT3-T4 or cN+). In this group of patients, the complete response rate was 79%, with 8 (42%) responders developing recurrence at a median of approximately 12 months, and 5-year overall and disease-free survival rates of 52% and 43%, respectively.[33] Others have also reported management of adenocarcinoma and squamous cell carcinoma with 5-fluorouracil and cisplatin and urothelial carcinoma with platinum-based poly-chemotherapeutic regimens.[34]

The utilization of mainly single modality radiation therapy has also been described in female patients with primary urothelial, squamous and adenocarcinoma of the urethra. The radiation treatment has involved external beam radiation alone, brachytherapy alone, or a combination of radiation modalities, utilizing 40 to 106 Gy of radiation. Selected patients have also received radiation to the regional lymph nodes. Reported local recurrence rates are 35% with this approach. Investigators reported a durable disease-free status in 38% of patients at median follow-up of 7.6 years, and another group reported a 5-year overall survival of 41%, with a local control rate of 64% at 5 years.[28,35–37]

SUMMARY

Recurrence of cancer in the urethra is a relatively uncommon clinical situation, whether metachronous following primary treatment(s) in other parts of the genitourinary tract or recurrence following treatment of primary urethral cancers. Initial detection of asymptomatic urethral recurrence depends on diligent clinical assessment with clinical and endoscopic examination or saline wash cytology. Although long-term outcomes in patients diagnosed with urethral recurrence by surveillance following cystectomy may not be different from those in patients presenting symptomatically, early detection of a more localized recurrence may afford the opportunity to explore less-invasive, potentially organ-preserving treatment options. Urethral recurrence in patients treated with radical cystectomy is relatively well documented, and both urethra-preserving and more surgically invasive management options are widely reported.

There is comparatively less evidence regarding the best management strategies in patients with relapse following treatment for primary urethral cancer, as the majority of information is extrapolated from experience with the actual primary tumors. Multimodal therapies should be considered in more advanced disease, as evidence from the management of patients with primary urethral cancer supports improved survival outcomes with multimodality approaches.

REFERENCES

1. Gakis G, Ali-El-Dein B, Babjuk M, et al. Urethral recurrence in women with orthotopic bladder substitutes: a multi-institutional study. Urol Oncol 2015; 33(5). 204.e17–23.
2. Soukup V, Babjuk M, Bellmunt J, et al. Follow-up after surgical treatment of bladder cancer: a critical analysis of the literature. Eur Urol 2012;62(2): 290–302.
3. Stenzl A, Draxl H, Posch B, et al. The risk of urethral tumors in female bladder cancer: can the urethra be used for orthotopic reconstruction of the lower urinary tract? J Urol 1995;153(3 Pt 2):950–5.
4. Yamashita S, Hoshi S, Ohyama C, et al. Urethral recurrence following neobladder in bladder cancer patients. Tohoku J Exp Med 2003;199(4):197–203.

5. Stenzl A, Bartsch G, Rogatsch H. The remnant urothelium after reconstructive bladder surgery. Eur Urol 2002;41(2):124–31.

6. Freeman JA, Tarter TA, Esrig D, et al. Urethral recurrence in patients with orthotopic ileal neobladders. J Urol 1996;156(5):1615–9.

7. Nieder AM, Sved PD, Gomez P, et al. Urethral recurrence after cystoprostatectomy: implications for urinary diversion and monitoring. Urology 2004;64(5):950–4.

8. Balci U, Dogantekin E, Ozer K, et al. Patterns, risks and outcomes of urethral recurrence after radical cystectomy for urothelial cancer; over 20 year single center experience. Int J Surg 2015;13:148–51.

9. Chan Y, Fisher P, Tilki D, et al. Urethral recurrence after cystectomy: current preventative measures, diagnosis and management. BJU Int 2016;117(4):563–9.

10. Mitra AP, Alemozaffar M, Harris BN, et al. Outcomes after urothelial recurrence in bladder cancer patients undergoing radical cystectomy. Urology 2014;84(6):1420–6.

11. Boorjian SA, Kim SP, Weight CJ, et al. Risk factors and outcomes of urethral recurrence following radical cystectomy. Eur Urol 2011;60(6):1266–72.

12. Stein JP, Clark P, Miranda G, et al. Urethral tumor recurrence following cystectomy and urinary diversion: clinical and pathological characteristics in 768 male patients. J Urol 2005;173(4):1163–8.

13. Varol C, Thalmann GN, Burkhard FC, et al. Treatment of urethral recurrence following radical cystectomy and ileal bladder substitution. J Urol 2004;172(3):937–42.

14. Lin DW, Herr HW, Dalbagni G. Value of urethral wash cytology in the retained male urethra after radical cystoprostatectomy. J Urol 2003;169(3):961–3.

15. Erckert M, Stenzl A, Falk M, et al. Incidence of urethral tumor involvement in 910 men with bladder cancer. World J Urol 1996;14(1):3–8.

16. Clark PE, Stein JP, Groshen SG, et al. The management of urethral transitional cell carcinoma after radical cystectomy for invasive bladder cancer. J Urol 2004;172(4 Pt 1):1342–7.

17. Huguet J, Monllau V, Sabate S, et al. Diagnosis, risk factors, and outcome of urethral recurrences following radical cystectomy for bladder cancer in 729 male patients. Eur Urol 2008;53(4):785–92 [discussion: 792–3].

18. Hrbacek J, Macek P, Ali-El-Dein B, et al. Treatment and outcomes of urethral recurrence of urinary bladder cancer in women after radical cystectomy and orthotopic neobladder: a series of 12 cases. Urol Int 2015;94(1):45–9.

19. Giannarini G, Kessler TM, Thoeny HC, et al. Do patients benefit from routine follow-up to detect recurrences after radical cystectomy and ileal orthotopic bladder substitution? Eur Urol 2010;58(4):486–94.

20. Yoshida K, Nishiyama H, Kinoshita H, et al. Surgical treatment for urethral recurrence after ileal neobladder reconstruction in patients with bladder cancer. BJU Int 2006;98(5):1008–11.

21. Miller MI, Benson MC. Management of urethral recurrence after radical cystectomy and neobladder creation by urethroscopic resection and fulguration. J Urol 1996;156(5):1768.

22. Leissner J, Stein R, Hohenfellner R, et al. Radical cystoprostatectomy combined with Mainz pouch bladder substitution to the urethra: long-term results. BJU Int 1999;83(9):964–70.

23. Akkad T, Gozzi C, Deibl M, et al. Tumor recurrence in the remnant urothelium of females undergoing radical cystectomy for transitional cell carcinoma of the bladder: long-term results from a single center. J Urol 2006;175(4):1268–71 [discussion: 1271].

24. Hakenberg OW, Franke HJ, Froehner M, et al. The treatment of primary urethral carcinoma–the dilemmas of a rare condition: experience with partial urethrectomy and adjuvant chemotherapy. Onkologie 2001;24(1):48–52.

25. Smith Y, Hadway P, Ahmed S, et al. Penile-preserving surgery for male distal urethral carcinoma. BJU Int 2007;100(1):82–7.

26. Davis JW, Schellhammer PF, Schlossberg SM. Conservative surgical therapy for penile and urethral carcinoma. Urology 1999;53(2):386–92.

27. Dalbagni G, Zhang ZF, Lacombe L, et al. Male urethral carcinoma: analysis of treatment outcome. Urology 1999;53(6):1126–32.

28. Dinney CP, Johnson DE, Swanson DA, et al. Therapy and prognosis for male anterior urethral carcinoma: an update. Urology 1994;43(4):506–14.

29. Dimarco DS, Dimarco CS, Zincke H, et al. Surgical treatment for local control of female urethral carcinoma. Urol Oncol 2004;22(5):404–9.

30. Karnes RJ, Breau RH, Lightner DJ. Surgery for urethral cancer. Urol Clin North Am 2010;37(3):445–57.

31. Gakis G, Witjes JA, Comperat E, et al. EAU guidelines on primary urethral carcinoma. Eur Urol 2013;64(5):823–30.

32. Dayyani F, Pettaway CA, Kamat AM, et al. Retrospective analysis of survival outcomes and the role of cisplatin-based chemotherapy in patients with urethral carcinomas referred to medical oncologists. Urol Oncol 2013;31(7):1171–7.

33. Kent M, Zinman L, Girshovich L, et al. Combined chemoradiation as primary treatment for invasive male urethral cancer. J Urol 2015;193(2):532–7.

34. Gheiler EL, Tefilli MV, Tiguert R, et al. Management of primary urethral cancer. Urology 1998;52(3): 487–93.

35. Dalbagni G, Zhang ZF, Lacombe L, et al. Female urethral carcinoma: an analysis of treatment outcome and a plea for a standardized management strategy. Br J Urol 1998;82(6):835–41.

36. Milosevic MF, Warde PR, Banerjee D, et al. Urethral carcinoma in women: results of treatment with primary radiotherapy. Radiother Oncol 2000;56(1): 29–35.

37. Garden AS, Zagars GK, Delclos L. Primary carcinoma of the female urethra. Results of radiation therapy. Cancer 1993;71(10):3102–8.

Preneoplastic and Primary Scrotal Cancer
Updates on Pathogenesis and Diagnostic Evaluation

CrossMark

Yao Zhu, MD, PhD[a,b], Ding-Wei Ye, MD, PhD[a,b],*

KEYWORDS

- Scrotal cancer
- Squamous cell carcinoma
- Extramammary Paget's disease
- Basal cell carcinoma

KEY POINTS

- Scrotal neoplasm has an annual incidence of approximately 1 per 1,000,000 males. Common histologic types are squamous cell carcinoma (SCC), extramammary Paget's disease (EMPD), and basal cell carcinoma (BCC).
- Scrotal SCC is not currently linked to occupational exposure. Oral psoralen and ultraviolet A photochemotherapy has been confirmed as carcinogenic factors.
- EMPD is classified into primary and secondary neoplasms. Scrotal EMPD is associated with an increased risk of gastrointestinal and genitourinary tumors.
- BCC in the scrotum has carcinogenic pathways other than sun exposure. Histologic classification of BCC is critical for prognosis and treatment.
- Diagnostic evaluation of scrotal cancer depends on pathologic subtypes. Inguinal lymph nodes are common metastatic sites in cases of invasive disease.

INTRODUCTION

The scrotum consists of skin, dartos muscle, and the external spermatic, cremaster, and internal spermatic fascia. The dermis of scrotal skin contains hair follicles and apocrine, eccrine, and sebaceous glands. Early in 1775, Pott[1] described a relationship between soot exposure and a high incidence of scrotal cancer among chimney sweepers. Since then, several occupational exposures have been causally linked to an increased risk of scrotal cancer. With this knowledge, primary preventative cares, including improved hygiene and avoidance of carcinogenic substances, have decreased remarkably the incidence of scrotal cancer. In the modern era, the incidence of scrotal malignancy is as low as 0.9 to 1.8 per 1,000,000 male persons per year.[2] The recent literature included reports

on more than 1000 cases of scrotal cancer. However, most of these lack accurate information that can be used for detailed assessment or are hypothesis-generating case reports. The rarity of cases and research impede our understanding of the changing diagram of scrotal cancer. Therefore, this article provides a summary of current knowledge, mainly focusing on pathogenesis and diagnostic evaluation, which may influence the prevention and early recognition of the disease.

PRENEOPLASTIC SQUAMOUS LESIONS AND SQUAMOUS CELL CARCINOMA
Pathogenesis

Bowen's disease and squamous cell carcinoma (SCC) are the most common histologic subtypes of scrotal neoplasm, accounting for 42% of all

[a] Department of Urology, Fudan University Shanghai Cancer Center, Shanghai, China; [b] Department of Oncology, Shanghai Medical College, Fudan University, No. 138 Yixueyuan Road, Shanghai 200032, China
* Corresponding author.
E-mail address: dwyeli@163.com

Urol Clin N Am 43 (2016) 523–530
http://dx.doi.org/10.1016/j.ucl.2016.06.013
0094-0143/16/© 2016 Elsevier Inc. All rights reserved.

cases in a population-based report from the Netherlands.[2] Historically, SCC was the first malignancy to be linked directly to exposure to occupational carcinogens. In addition to soot, SCC has also been linked to exposure to tar, pith, different types of lubricating and cutting oils, creosotes, gas production, and paraffin wax pressing. Owing to the substantial improvements in working environments, occupational risk factors have not been associated with increased risk of scrotal SCC in the last 2 decades.[3]

Ultraviolet exposure is a well-known risk factor for skin cancer. A nationwide population-based case control study found a near significantly increased risk (odds ratio [OR], 6.7; 95% CI, 1.0–45.6) for scrotal SCC with a cumulative lifetime duration of nude sunbathing of 26 to 150 hours.[4] In addition, the results suggested that the use of sunbeds seemed to increase the risk of scrotal SCC (OR, 3.2; 95% CI, 1.0–10.4). Moreover, iatrogenic ultraviolet radiation for skins diseases was associated with a remarkably high risk of scrotal SCC. In a cohort of men with psoriasis who had been treated with oral psoralen and ultraviolet A photochemotherapy (PUVA) and followed for 12.3 years, Stern and colleagues[5] found a risk ratio of 95.7 (95% CI, 43.8–181.8) for genital SCC in treated patients compared with population incidence data. Notably, the mean age of patients treated with PUVA was 46 years, which is significantly lower than the mean age in sporadic cases (65 in the Surveillance, Epidemiology, and End Results database[6]). The carcinogenic effect of PUVA was also dose dependent: in patients exposed to high levels of PUVA, the incidence of invasive SCC was 16.3 times (95% CI, 9.4–26.4) that of patients exposed to low levels. With a further 10 years of follow-up, Stern and colleagues[7] found a 52.6-fold (95% CI, 19.3–114.6) increase in the incidence of genital SCCs in this cohort compared with that expected for the general white population. Although most of the cohort patients had stopped PUVA treatment or used genital shielding since first publication, long-term follow-up showed a constant incidence of genital tumors after treatment stopped and indicated that PUVA presents a persistent risk. Conversely, the link between PUVA and SCC was not confirmed in European prospective studies with relatively short follow-up periods.[8] However, analysis of a large population-based database with an observation period of at least 14 years showed a relative risk of 5.6 to 6.5 for SCC in European men.[9,10] The male genitalia seem to be more susceptible to the carcinogenic effects of PUVA than nongenital areas. In the PUVA Follow-Up study, genital tumors comprised 3.3% of all invasive and in situ SCCs. In the general population, genital tumors comprised only 0.2% of all nonmelanoma skin cancers. The carcinogenic effects of the PUVA therapy include DNA damage accumulation and immunosuppression.[11] No increased risk of skin cancer has been reported in studies assessing the carcinogenic risk of narrowband UVB, which is used now more commonly for treating psoriasis.[12]

Human papillomavirus (HPV) was previously linked to scrotal SCC in a study of 14 patients at the Mayo Clinic.[13] Out of a 14 total cases, 6 (42%) had a history and histologic evidence of HPV infection. Matoso and colleagues evaluated a total of 29 cases of SCC of the scrotum in 3 North American institutions occurring between 1999 and 2013. Of 26 cases with available tissue, 7 (27%) tested positive for high-risk HPV serotypes using in situ hybridization. Cases associated with HPV-infected disease displayed a predominantly basaloid or warty morphology and were characterized by p16 and Ki-67 immunostaining. Similar morphologic and immunohistochemical results in HPV-infected patients suggested similar a pathogenic pathway proposed for penile SCC.[14] Furthermore, scrotal SCC may be a manifestation of cutaneous carcinoma risk in immunodeficient patients. Matoso and colleagues[15] found that 5 of 29 patients with SCC of the scrotum had immune compromised conditions such as with infection with the human immunodeficiency virus, after transplantation, and in leukemia.

Diagnostic Evaluation

Scrotal SCC lesions present as slow-growing plaques, nodules, or ulcerations. Advanced disease may invade the testes or penis. The diagnosis is confirmed by histologic evaluation, and several areas should be sampled to determine the boundary of extension and depth of invasion. The most commonly used staging system is the Lowe modification of the system proposed by Ray and Whoitmore.[16] It is based on the extent of local disease and the level of metastasis (Table 1). The scrotum has the same lymphatic drainage pattern as the penis. Tumors usually spread stepwise from the inguinal lymph nodes to the pelvic lymph nodes. Interestingly, the scrotal lymphatics do not cross the median raphe and drain into the ipsilateral superficial inguinal lymph nodes. Therefore, tumors without involvement of the median raphe rarely metastasize to the opposite inguinal site.[17] Because of similarities in location and histology, the clinical workup of scrotal SCC is quite similar to that of penile cancer. Routine imaging examinations included pelvic/abdominal computed tomography (CT) scans and chest radiographs. Other tests such as chest

Table 1
Diagnostic evaluation in scrotal squamous cell carcinoma in according to tumor stage

Staging Category	Description	Key Points	Approaches
A1	Disease localized to the scrotum	Lesion boundary, multifocal and depth of invasion	Physical examination, multiple biopsy
A2	Locally extensive tumor invading adjacent structures	Plan of surgery, inform of removal of other organ	Physical examination, imaging, diagnostic biopsy
B	Metastatic disease involving inguinal lymph nodes only	Microscopic inguinal lymph node metastases	Sentinel lymph node biopsy, lymph node dissection
C	Metastatic disease involving pelvic lymph nodes without evidence of distant spread	Microscopic pelvic lymph node metastases	Lymph node dissection, PET-CT scan
D	Metastasis beyond the pelvic lymph nodes to involve distant organs	Suspicious lesions	PET-CT scan, diagnostic biopsy

From Lowe FC. Squamous cell carcinoma of the scrotum. J Urol 1983;130(3):423–7; with permission.

CT and bone scans are used when indicated. Physical examination and cross-sectional imaging techniques are inaccurate for determining lymph node metastasis in cases of invasive scrotal SCC.[18] An inflammatory reaction may cause enlargement of the inguinal lymph nodes and fine-needle aspiration cytology is the easiest way to confirm metastasis. However, the examination is only helpful if the results are positive. If the fine-needle aspiration cytology is negative and a lymph node is still palpable after antibiotic treatment, an excision biopsy is advised. In cases of clinically negative inguinal nodal basin, approximately 23% of patients will harbor occult metastases.[19,20] Unfortunately, ultrasound with fine-needle aspiration cytology reportedly failed to identify 35% of inguinal basins with metastatic lymph nodes.[20] On the contrary, the addition of dynamic sentinel lymph node biopsy (SLNB) improved the detection rate to 95% and can serve as an alternative to prophylactic lymph node dissection in dedicated centers.[20] For pelvic lymph node metastases, PET-CT scan reportedly showed a sensitivity of 91%, a specificity of 100%, and a diagnostic accuracy of 96% in a pilot study of 28 pelvic basins.[21] The imaging technique, however, should be replicated in the venues of a large prospective cohort and hence at the present time cannot replace surgery as the standard staging approach.

EXTRAMAMMARY PAGET'S DISEASE
Pathogenesis

Extramammary Paget's disease (EMPD) is an adenocarcinoma that is found mostly on apocrine gland-bearing skin such as the scrotum, penis, vulva and anus. The cell origin of EMPD remains controversial, and the pathogenesis is still the subject of great debate. Mammary Paget's disease (MPD) is associated with an underlying breast cancer in 92% to 100% of cases, and the main explanation for MPD is epidermotropic spread, in which tumor cells originating from the underlying mammary carcinoma migrate via the lactiferous ducts and invade the epidermis of the nipple and areola. EMPD is associated less commonly with an underlying adnexal or distant carcinoma. The probability of internal malignancy ranges from 45% in perianal EMPD to 11% in genital EMPD.[22] Current evidence suggests that EMPD is a heterogeneous disease and Wilkinson and Brown[23] have proposed a classification system based on the origin of neoplastic Paget cells (**Box 1**).

Primary Paget's disease is proposed to originate from pluripotent keratinocyte stem cells.[24] It has also been suggested that Toker cells are precursors of EMPD. Toker cells, found in 10% of normal nipples, have been thought to be the precursor of MPD since 1970.[25] Examinations of the histologic and ultrastructural features of the cells of EMPD and Toker cells suggest that these are benign and malignant counterparts.[26] Willman and colleagues[27] examined 11 vulvectomies and found the presence of Toker cells in 4 (36%) of the vulvar samples. Therefore, the presence of Toker cells with mammarylike glands of the genital skin suggested that EMPD could develop in a manner similar to primary MPD.[28] Less commonly, EMPD is an epidermal manifestation of an underlying skin neoplasm, usually a tumor of the apocrine or eccrine glands.

Secondary EMPD, by contrast, results from the epidermotropic spread or metastasis of an underlying internal malignancy, commonly a genitourinary or gastrointestinal carcinoma. Secondary EMPD lesions may have similar immunohistochemical profiles as the visceral lesions.[29]

Finally, a multicentric pathogenetic approach had been suggested, in which an oncogenic stimulus induces both the EMPD and the underlying (adnexal or visceral) tumor. This theory explains the existence of multiple forms of EMPD, as well as the rare associations between MPD and EMPD.

Diagnostic Evaluation

EMPD accounts for approximately 20% of scrotal neoplasms and is commonly found in the Asian population.[6,30] Clinically, EMPD typically presents as erythematous plaques with pruritus, pain, or oozing. Approximately 29% of cases have the appearance of depigmentation with grey-white patches. The mean age of men with scrotal EMPD is approximately 70 years old.[6,31] However, the disease may be misdiagnosed clinically as eczema or dermatitis, which may delay pathologic examination.[32]

Diagnostic evaluation of EMPD includes 3 parts: histologic classification, search for underlying visceral disease, and defining extent of involvement (**Fig. 1**). The first 2 parts are used to establish the EMPD disease category, and the last part is used to define treatment and prognosis. **Table 2** summarizes the probability and common types of internal malignancies in scrotal EMPD.[30–36] The percentage with internal malignancies is higher in the Western population compared with Asian counterparts. Interestingly, the location of internal tumors also seems to differ between Western and Eastern ethnic groups.

Intraepithelial EMPD rarely metastases, but invasive disease may spread to regional lymphatics and other organs such as bones, liver, and lungs.[37,38] Zhu and colleagues[37] compared the clinicopathologic features of metastatic and nonmetastatic penoscrotal EMPD. They found that dermal or deeper invasion and lymphovascular embolization were strong predictors of metastasis. In a large

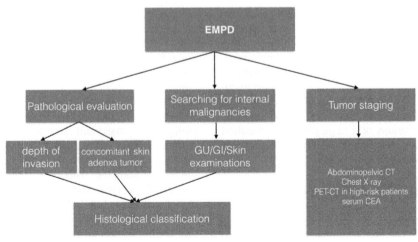

Fig. 1. The paradigm of diagnostic evaluation of scrotal extramammary Paget's disease (EMPD). CEA, carcinoembryonic antigen; CT, computed tomography; GI, gastrointestinal; GU, genitourinary.

Table 2
Literature review of the probability and common types of internal malignancy in male genital extramammary Paget's disease

Author, Year	Countries	n	Age, y (Mean)	Percentage with Internal Malignancies[b]		
				Overall, %	GU, %	GI, %
Lai et al,[33] 2003	China	33	68.6	9.1	6.1	3
Choi et al,[34] 2005	Korea	31	62.2	29	3.2	22.6
Zhu et al,[32] 2007	China	38	73[a]	7.9	0	2.6
Lee et al,[36] 2011	Korea	129 scrotal	67.5	14.4	0	9.4
Kang et al,[31] 2015	China	211	63.9	6.2	1.4	2.8
Hegarty et al,[35] 2011	US	20	50–86	45	30	10
Herrel et al,[30] 2014	US	237 penoscrotal	71.9	47.1	—	—

Abbreviations: GI, gastrointestinal; GU, genitourinary.
[a] Median.
[b] Criteria to define associated internal malignancies varied among these studies.

series of 145 patients with EMPD, Ito and co-workers[39] reported probabilities of lymph node metastasis of 15.4% and 34.8% in tumor invasion of the papillary and reticular dermis, respectively. These findings were confirmed further in other pilot studies and together prompt a thorough clinical workup in high-risk patients.[38,40,41] Compared with conventional imaging modalities, fludeoxyglucose PET-CT scanning demonstrated high sensitivity in detecting occult metastatic lesions.[37,42] In a small series of 10 cases, Tian and colleagues[42] found that 20.4% of detected lymph nodes were smaller than 1 cm in diameter with an average maximum standardized uptake value of 4. Except for lung metastases, large lymph nodes and other visceral metastases had high standardized uptake value uptake (6–7). Overall, 3 of 10 patients were upstaged using PET-CT. In a large Japanese cohort, SLNB was evaluated for staging of inguinal lymph nodes in invasive EMPD.[43] In a total of 107 patients without clinical lymphadenopathy, SLNB was able to identify 16 patients (15%) with occult metastatic disease. However, 7 of 91 patients without sentinel lymph node metastasis subsequently developed lymph node relapse in the follow-up. Overall, SLNB achieved a moderate detection rate of 69.6% (16 of 23) in clinical node-negative patients. Among those patients with elevated serum carcinoembryonic antigen at diagnosis, the marker can be used to monitor tumor progression.[37]

BASAL CELL CARCINOMA
Pathogenesis

Exposure to ultraviolet radiation is the major risk factor associated with the development of BCC.[44] BCC commonly occurs in body areas exposed to the sun, such as the head and neck (80% of cases) and is rarely found in sun protected area. Only 121 genital BCCs were reported in a 33-year span from Surveillance, Epidemiology, and End Results databases.[6] The predisposing factors for BCC in areas not exposed to the sun are still unclear. Gibson and colleagues[45] found 17 of 51 patients (36%) with perianal and genital BC had a history of nonmelanoma skin cancer in sun-exposed areas. Their findings indicated that one-third of genital SCC tumors share the same carcinogenic pathway as those in common areas. Other risk factors, such as immunosuppression status, previous radiation, and chronic skin irritation, may also play a role in the development of scrotal SCC. In a nationwide case-control study, Verhoeven and colleagues[4] reported that scrotal BCC may be related to previous cancer diagnoses. Gibson and colleagues[45] reported that 8.5% of perianal and genital BCC cases had a history of radiotherapy in the pelvic region. Dai and colleagues[46] reviewed 10 cases of scrotal BCC and found a common history of poor sanitation and local chronic skin inflammation.

Diagnostic Evaluation

To diagnose BCC, a skin biopsy is performed for histopathologic evaluation. Based on growth patterns, BCC can be divided into subgroups, such as nodular, superficial, infiltrative, micronodular, morpheiform, and so on. In a large retrospective series of 1039 consecutive BCCs, 21% were nodular, 17.4% were superficial, 14.5% were micronodular, 7.4% were infiltrative, and 1.1% were morpheiform.[47] Roughly one-third of tumors showed a mixed histologic patterns. The histologic spectrum of BCC impacts treatment and prognosis.[48] The indolent growth variants include nodular and superficial BCC. The aggressive growth BCCs are infiltrative, metatypical, and morpheiform or sclerosing BCC. In a recent report of 10 scrotal BCC cases, 2 patients had an aggressive growth pattern and developed metastatic disease during follow-up.[46]

BCC commonly grows slowly and metastasis is rare. The metastatic rate reported in the literature ranges from 0.0028% to 0.55%.[49] The most commonly reported metastatic sites are the lymph nodes, lungs, and bones.[50] The median duration between the onset of the primary disease and the occurrence of metastasis was 6 years.[50] Thus far, of the 53 reported scrotal BCC cases, 7 patients (13.2%) developed metastasis 2 to 4 years after initial treatment of the primary lesion.[46,51] The most common metastatic sites were the inguinal lymph nodes, which were present in 4 of 7 cases. Therefore, routine evaluation of the inguinal nodal basin is recommended in the diagnostic evaluation of scrotal BCC.

SUMMARY

Scrotal neoplasm is a rare disease with an annual incidence of approximately 1 per 1,000,000 males. Pathogenesis and diagnostic evaluation greatly depend on the disease's histology type. Currently, scrotal SCC is not linked to occupational exposure as reported in historical series. Prospective studies have confirmed PUVA as a strong carcinogenic factor for SCC. EMPD is classified into primary and secondary neoplasms according to the presence of concomitant internal malignancies. Scrotal EMPD is associated with an increased risk of gastrointestinal and genitourinary tumors. BCC in the scrotum has a carcinogenic pathway other than sun exposure. Histologic stratification of BCC into indolent and aggressive variants is critical for determining prognosis and treatment. Generally, the inguinal lymph nodes have been common metastatic sites in cases of invasive disease.

REFERENCES

1. Pott P. Chirurgical observations relative to the cataract, the polypus of the nose, the cancer of the scrotum, the different kinds of ruptures, and the mortification of the toes and feet. London: Hawes, Clarke and Collins; 1775.
2. Verhoeven RH, Louwman WJ, Koldewijn EL, et al. Scrotal cancer: incidence, survival and second primary tumours in the Netherlands since 1989. Br J Cancer 2010;103(9):1462–6.
3. Verhoeven RH, Kiemeney LA, Coebergh JW, et al. Occupation and scrotal cancer: results of the NOCCA study. Acta Oncol 2011;50(8):1244–6.
4. Verhoeven RH, Aben KK, van Rossum MM, et al. New insights into the aetiology of scrotal cancer, a nationwide case-control study in the Netherlands. J Eur Acad Dermatol Venereol 2014;28(1):65–71.
5. Stern RS. Genital tumors among men with psoriasis exposed to psoralens and ultraviolet A radiation (PUVA) and ultraviolet B radiation. The Photochemotherapy Follow-up Study. N Engl J Med 1990;322(16):1093–7.
6. Johnson TV, Hsiao W, Delman KA, et al. Scrotal cancer survival is influenced by histology: a SEER study. World J Urol 2013;31(3):585–90.
7. Stern RS, Bagheri S, Nichols K, et al. The persistent risk of genital tumors among men treated with psoralen plus ultraviolet A (PUVA) for psoriasis. J Am Acad Dermatol 2002;47(1):33–9.
8. Henseler T, Christophers E, Honigsmann H, et al. Skin tumors in the European PUVA Study. Eight-year follow-up of 1,643 patients treated with PUVA for psoriasis. J Am Acad Dermatol 1987;16(1 Pt 1):108–16.
9. Lindelof B, Sigurgeirsson B, Tegner E, et al. PUVA and cancer risk: the Swedish follow-up study. Br J Dermatol 1999;141(1):108–12.
10. Hannuksela-Svahn A, Pukkala E, Laara E, et al. Psoriasis, its treatment, and cancer in a cohort of Finnish patients. J Invest Dermatol 2000;114(3):587–90.
11. Matsumura Y, Ananthaswamy HN. Toxic effects of ultraviolet radiation on the skin. Toxicol Appl Pharmacol 2004;195(3):298–308.
12. Archier E, Devaux S, Castela E, et al. Carcinogenic risks of psoralen UV-A therapy and narrowband UV-B therapy in chronic plaque psoriasis: a systematic literature review. J Eur Acad Dermatol Venereol 2012;26(Suppl 3):22–31.
13. Andrews PE, Farrow GM, Oesterling JE. Squamous cell carcinoma of the scrotum: long-term followup of 14 patients. J Urol 1991;146(5):1299–304.
14. Ferreux E, Lont AP, Horenblas S, et al. Evidence for at least three alternative mechanisms targeting the p16INK4A/cyclin D/Rb pathway in penile carcinoma, one of which is mediated by high-risk human papillomavirus. J Pathol 2003;201(1):109–18.
15. Matoso A, Ross HM, Chen S, et al. Squamous neoplasia of the scrotum: a series of 29 cases. Am J Surg Pathol 2014;38(7):973–81.
16. Lowe FC. Squamous cell carcinoma of the scrotum. J Urol 1983;130(3):423–7.
17. Chung BI, Sommer G, Brooks JD. Surgical, radiology, and endoscopic anatomy of the male pelvis. In: Wein AJ, Kavoussi LR, Partin AW, et al, editors. Campbell-Walsh urology tenth edition, vol. 3. Philadelphia: Elsevier; 2015. p. 1630.
18. Hughes B, Leijte J, Shabbir M, et al. Non-invasive and minimally invasive staging of regional lymph

nodes in penile cancer. World J Urol 2009;27(2): 197–203.

19. Zhu Y, Zhang HL, Yao XD, et al. Development and evaluation of a nomogram to predict inguinal lymph node metastasis in patients with penile cancer and clinically negative lymph nodes. J Urol 2010; 184(2):539–45.

20. Lam W, Alnajjar HM, La-Touche S, et al. Dynamic sentinel lymph node biopsy in patients with invasive squamous cell carcinoma of the penis: a prospective study of the long-term outcome of 500 inguinal basins assessed at a single institution. Eur Urol 2013;63(4):657–63.

21. Graafland NM, Leijte JA, Valdes Olmos RA, et al. Scanning with 18F-FDG-PET/CT for detection of pelvic nodal involvement in inguinal node-positive penile carcinoma. Eur Urol 2009;56(2):339–45.

22. Kanitakis J. Mammary and extramammary Paget's disease. J Eur Acad Dermatol Venereol 2007;21(5): 581–90.

23. Wilkinson EJ, Brown HM. Vulvar Paget disease of urothelial origin: a report of three cases and a proposed classification of vulvar Paget disease. Hum Pathol 2002;33(5):549–54.

24. Lloyd J, Flanagan AM. Mammary and extramammary Paget's disease. J Clin Pathol 2000;53(10):742–9.

25. Toker C. Clear cells of the nipple epidermis. Cancer 1970;25(3):601–10.

26. Marucci G, Betts CM, Golouh R, et al. Toker cells are probably precursors of Paget cell carcinoma: a morphological and ultrastructural description. Virchows Arch 2002;441(2):117–23.

27. Willman JH, Golitz LE, Fitzpatrick JE. Vulvar clear cells of Toker: precursors of extramammary Paget's disease. Am J Dermatopathol 2005;27(3): 185–8.

28. Belousova IE, Kazakov DV, Michal M, et al. Vulvar Toker cells: the long-awaited missing link: a proposal for an origin-based histogenetic classification of extramammary Paget disease. Am J Dermatopathol 2006;28(1):84–6.

29. Brown HM, Wilkinson EJ. Uroplakin-III to distinguish primary vulvar Paget disease from Paget disease secondary to urothelial carcinoma. Hum Pathol 2002;33(5):545–8.

30. Herrel LA, Weiss AD, Goodman M, et al. Extramammary Paget's disease in males: survival outcomes in 495 patients. Ann Surg Oncol 2015; 22(5):1625–30.

31. Kang Z, Zhang Q, Zhang Q, et al. Clinical and pathological characteristics of extramammary Paget's disease: report of 246 Chinese male patients. Int J Clin Exp Pathol 2015;8(10):13233–40.

32. Zhu Y, Ye DW, Chen ZW, et al. Frozen sectionguided wide local excision in the treatment of penoscrotal extramammary Paget's disease. BJU Int 2007;100(6):1282–7.

33. Lai YL, Yang WG, Tsay PK, et al. Penoscrotal extramammary Paget's disease: a review of 33 cases in a 20-year experience. Plast Reconstr Surg 2003; 112(4):1017–23.

34. Choi YD, Cho NH, Park YS, et al. Lymphovascular and marginal invasion as useful prognostic indicators and the role of c-erbB-2 in patients with male extramammary Paget's disease: a study of 31 patients. J Urol 2005;174(2):561–5.

35. Hegarty PK, Suh J, Fisher MB, et al. Penoscrotal extramammary Paget's disease: the University of Texas M. D. Anderson Cancer Center contemporary experience. J Urol 2011;186(1):97–102.

36. Lee SJ, Choe YS, Jung HD, et al. A multicenter study on extramammary Paget's disease in Korea. Int J Dermatol 2011;50(5):508–15.

37. Zhu Y, Ye DW, Yao XD, et al. Clinicopathological characteristics, management and outcome of metastatic penoscrotal extramammary Paget's disease. Br J Dermatol 2009;161(3):577–82.

38. Dai B, Kong YY, Chang K, et al. Primary invasive carcinoma associated with penoscrotal extramammary Paget's disease: a clinicopathological analysis of 56 cases. BJU Int 2015;115(1):153–60.

39. Ito T, Kaku Y, Nagae K, et al. Tumor thickness as a prognostic factor in extramammary Paget's disease. J Dermatol 2015;42(3):269–75.

40. Yamada Y, Matsumoto T, Arakawa A, et al. Evaluation using a combination of lymphatic invasion on D2-40 immunostain and depth of dermal invasion is a strong predictor for nodal metastasis in extramammary Paget's disease. Pathol Int 2008; 58(2):114–7.

41. Shiomi T, Noguchi T, Nakayama H, et al. Clinicopathological study of invasive extramammary Paget's disease: subgroup comparison according to invasion depth. J Eur Acad Dermatol Venereol 2013; 27(5):589–92.

42. Tian Y, Wu HB, Li DL, et al. Utility of 18F-FDG PET/CT in the diagnosis and staging of extramammary Paget's disease. Nucl Med Commun 2015; 36(9):892–7.

43. Fujisawa Y, Yoshino K, Kiyohara Y, et al. The role of sentinel lymph node biopsy in the management of invasive extramammary Paget's disease: multicenter, retrospective study of 151 patients. J Dermatol Sci 2015;79(1):38–42.

44. Rubin AI, Chen EH, Ratner D. Basal-cell carcinoma. N Engl J Med 2005;353(21):2262–9.

45. Gibson GE, Ahmed I. Perianal and genital basal cell carcinoma: A clinicopathologic review of 51 cases. J Am Acad Dermatol 2001;45(1):68–71.

46. Dai B, Kong YY, Ye DW, et al. Basal cell carcinoma of the scrotum: clinicopathologic analysis of 10 cases. Dermatol Surg 2012;38(5):783–90.

47. Sexton M, Jones DB, Maloney ME. Histologic pattern analysis of basal cell carcinoma. Study of a

series of 1039 consecutive neoplasms. J Am Acad Dermatol 1990;23(6 Pt 1):1118–26.

48. Crowson AN. Basal cell carcinoma: biology, morphology and clinical implications. Mod Pathol 2006;19(Suppl 2):S127–47.

49. Ganti AK, Kessinger A. Systemic therapy for disseminated basal cell carcinoma: an uncommon manifestation of a common cancer. Cancer Treat Rev 2011;37(6):440–3.

50. McCusker M, Basset-Seguin N, Dummer R, et al. Metastatic basal cell carcinoma: prognosis dependent on anatomic site and spread of disease. Eur J Cancer 2014;50(4):774–83.

51. Kinoshita R, Yamamoto O, Yasuda H, et al. Basal cell carcinoma of the scrotum with lymph node metastasis: report of a case and review of the literature. Int J Dermatol 2005; 44(1):54–6.

Surgical Management of Primary Scrotal Cancer

Jonathan H. Huang, MD*, Matt Broggi, MSc, Adeboye O. Osunkoya, MD,
Viraj A. Master, MD, PhD

KEYWORDS

- Scrotal cancer • Squamous cell carcinoma • Extramammary Paget's disease • Sarcoma
- Basal cell carcinoma • Melanoma • Adnexal skin tumor

KEY POINTS

- Wide surgical excision is recommended for localized scrotal cancer.
- Reconstruction of the defect can be performed with primary closure, skin grafts, or flaps.
- High-risk scrotal cancer has a poor prognosis, with a decreased overall survival compared with penile cancer.

INTRODUCTION

Percival Pott, the 18th-century English surgeon, is credited as the first to associate an occupational exposure to the ensuing development of disease.[1] Cases of squamous cell carcinoma of the scrotum, known colloquially as chimney sweep's carcinoma, were seen almost exclusively in England among young men who worked as chimney sweepers.[2] Sweeps, as they were called, were forced to work in dirty conditions and many times worked while naked to fit into tight spaces. This led to the overexposure of coal on the genitals and the subsequent development of soot warts and cancer, if left untreated. More recently, polycyclic aromatic hydrocarbons in the soot were discovered to be the causative agent of this disease and steps were taken to protect workers.[3] As occupational exposure has decreased, so has the incidence of scrotal cancer, which makes studying this virulent malignancy much more difficult.

Primary scrotal cancers are rare, with the majority of the literature being composed of small case series. Johnson and colleagues[4] evaluated the Surveillance, Epidemiology, and End Results database for scrotal cancer patients and found that histologies included squamous cell carcinoma (35.1%), extramammary Paget's disease (21.9%),

sarcoma (20.4%), basal cell carcinoma (16.7%), melanoma (3.3%), and adnexal skin tumors (2.6%). The median (95% CI) overall survival for localized low-risk scrotal cancers (basal cell carcinoma, extramammary Paget's disease, sarcoma) and localized high-risk scrotal cancers (melanoma, squamous cell carcinoma, adnexal skin tumors) was 166 (145–188) and 118 (101–135) months, respectively. Patients with regional and distant disease are reported to have worse overall survival.[5,6]

Diagnosis requires an excisional biopsy of the lesions to determine the underlying histology of the scrotal cancer. Evaluation of nonlocalized disease and metastases can be performed through careful physical examination and cross-sectional imaging modalities such as computed tomography scanning or MRI. PET should be regarded as investigational. Treatment for all histologies requires surgical removal of the malignancy. Adjuvant treatments, including radiation and chemotherapy may be warranted. Owing to the small number of reported cases, details in management and overall prognosis are limited. We discuss surgical management of primary scrotal cancers based on National Comprehensive Cancer Network guidelines, if present, and also expert opinion (**Box 1**).

Department of Urology, Emory University, 1365 Clifton Road Northeast, Suite B6140, Atlanta, GA 30322, USA
* Corresponding author.
E-mail address: jhhuan2@emory.edu

Urol Clin N Am 43 (2016) 531–544
http://dx.doi.org/10.1016/j.ucl.2016.06.014

TECHNIQUE/PROCEDURE
Preparation

Scrotal anatomy
The skin of the scrotum can be divided into an anterior and a posterior aspect, each with distinct neurovasculature. The anterior scrotum is supplied by the deep external pudendal arteries, which branch off the femoral artery and course medially into the scrotum. The posterior scrotum is supplied by the perineal arteries, which branch off the pudendal arteries. The vessels do not cross the median raphe and this allows for a relatively bloodless incision.

The anterior scrotal skin and the posterior scrotal skin have their own dedicated venous drainage that course along with their respective arterial supplies. The anterior surface is drained via the external pudendal veins and the posterior surface by the scrotal branches of the perineal vessels. The lymphatic drainage of the scrotum is supplied by the superficial inguinal lymph nodes for both the anterior and posterior sides. This differs from testicular lymphatics, which drain into the paraortic lymph nodes. The innervation of the scrotal skin is provided by the anterior scrotal nerves, which are branches of the ilioinguinal nerve, and the posterior scrotal nerves, which are branches of the perineal nerve.

Preoperative prophylactic antibiotic and infection management
The American Urologic Association best practice policy guidelines on surgical antimicrobial prophylaxis of the scrotum recommends a single dose of preoperative antibiotics, particularly in patients with certain risk factors for infection (**Table 1**).[7] This is owing, in part, to the scrotal surgical infection rate being comparatively low, ranging from 0% to 10%. The recommended prophylactic antibiotic of choice is a first-generation cephalosporin or clindamycin as an alternative.

Traditionally, hair has been removed preoperatively to reduce the risk of surgical site infections, although recent studies indicated that this may not be necessary. A recent analysis of randomized, controlled trials compared hair removal with no removal, the different methods of hair removal, as well as the different times of hair removal before surgery.[8] No significant difference in surgical site infections was found among patients who had their hair removed and those who did not. In circumstances when removal of hair is necessary, using clippers instead of a razor is associated with fewer surgical site infections.

Patient Positioning

1. The patient should be placed in the exaggerated dorsal lithotomy position to provide visualization of the entire scrotum and adjacent regions, including the penis, suprapubic/inguinal regions, medial thigh, and perineum/perianal regions.

Table 1
Factors and results

Factor	Result
Impaired natural defense mechanism	

Advanced age
   Anatomic anomalies of the urinary tract
   Poor nutritional status
   Smoking
   Chronic corticosteroid use
   Immunodeficiency
	Decreased natural defense mechanisms of the urinary tract and immune system

Increase local bacterial concentration and/or spectrum of flora	

Externalized catheters
   Colonized endogenous/exogenous material
   Distant coexistent infection
   Prolonged hospitalization
	Increased local bacterial concentration and/or spectrum

2. Betadine scrub and paint can be used to widely prepare the scrotum and adjacent regions.
3. Towels should be placed in a triangular manner around the scrotum. The penis can be reflected cephalad, covered by the towel over the suprapubic region. During the case, the towels can be adjusted to access adjacent region, if necessary. Standard cystoscopy drapes can be used.

Approach

General thoughts regarding surgical excision

- Scrotal cancer most often presents superficially. The skin and dartos of the scrotum is thicker than the respective tissue in the penis, which contributes to the superficial nature of this disease
- As with any surgery for resectable malignancy, the goal is to remove the disease with clear margins (both peripheral and deep). Mohs surgery and frozen sections can be used to ensure adequate margins.

General thoughts regarding reconstruction

- The scrotal skin is extremely elastic, which helps to provide coverage for reconstruction. Factors that contribute to a larger scrotum include older age and men with hydroceles.
- Approximately 60% of the scrotal skin can be removed with adequate tissue remaining for primary closure. Primary closure is preferred over skin grafts or flaps when possible.
- Closed suction drains can be considered to prevent the development of fluids collections, such as seromas and hematomas.

Technique and Procedure (Detailed Steps)

The goal of surgical treatment for scrotal cancer is excision of the disease. We present steps in management for the various histologic subtypes of scrotal cancer. We also present a case of scrotal cancer diagnosed at our institution, along with pictures taken during the surgery and reconstruction.

Squamous cell carcinoma

1. Biopsy-proven lesions should be excised with 4- to 6-mm clinical margins. Mohs surgery can alternatively be performed.[9]
2. Margins should be assessed. If positive, surgical reexcision should be performed. If unable to obtain a negative margin, which would be rare, radiation therapy is recommended.
3. Fine needle aspiration or core biopsy should be performed for palpable regional lymph nodes or abnormal lymph nodes identified on imaging. If positive and operable, regional lymph node dissection should be performed. Radiation therapy should be considered if multiple lymph nodes are involved or if extracapsular extension is present. If regional lymph nodes are positive and inoperable, radiation therapy with or without systemic therapy is recommended.
4. Excision site can be managed with tension-free primary approximation, skin graft, or flap and, seldom, with healing by secondary intention.
5. Nonsurgical candidates should receive radiation therapy.
6. Minimal evidence is available regarding systemic therapy for metastatic disease.

Extramammary Paget's disease

1. Biopsy-proven lesions should be excised with a wide surgical margin and intraoperative frozen section to ensure complete resection.[10]
2. The excision site can be managed with primary closure. A simultaneous reconstructive procedure, including a skin graft or flap, can be performed if the defect is unable to be closed primarily.
3. Imiquimod cream, 5-fluorouracil cream, and CO_2 laser have been used with variable results. Photodynamic therapy has been used for palliative results.
4. Of note, traditionally extramammary Paget's disease was thought to represent adenocarcinoma in situ, arising from the epidermis. However, more advanced disease, including deeper invasion, nodal disease, and metastatic disease have been reported, with 1 large series reporting up to 16.6% of patients with regional or distant disease.[5] Although the role of radiation therapy and chemotherapy is not entirely clear, these modalities have been applied as primary treatment, as adjuvant therapy, and for nonsurgical candidates. It is important to assess for other malignancies, because there may be an association with other underlying malignancies in patients with extramammary Paget's disease.

Sarcoma

1. Biopsy-proven lesions are treated according to stage.[11]
   A. For stage I sarcoma, wide local excisional surgery should be performed to obtain adequate negative oncologic margins. Although an adequate margin size is not specified, close margins may be necessary to preserve critical neurovascular and musculoskeletal structures. Failure to obtain adequate oncologic margins can be

managed by re-resection or radiation therapy.

B. For stage IIA sarcoma that is resectable with functional outcomes, surgery, surgery with adjuvant radiation, or neoadjuvant radiation therapy with surgery can be performed.

C. For stage IIB and III sarcomas that are resectable with functional outcomes, surgery, neoadjuvant radiation therapy and surgery, neoadjuvant chemoradiation and surgery, or neoadjuvant chemotherapy and surgery can be performed. Adjuvant radiation therapy with or without chemotherapy can be given.

D. For stage II and III sarcomas that are resectable with adverse functional outcomes or unresectable disease, radiation therapy, chemoradiation, chemotherapy, or regional limb therapy can be performed. If the lesion is subsequently resectable with acceptable functional outcomes, surgery should be performed. Adjuvant radiation therapy with or without chemotherapy can be performed.

E. For nodal involvement, regional lymph node dissection should be performed with or without radiation and chemotherapy.

F. For metastatic disease to a single organ and limited tumor bulk that is amenable to local therapy, metastasectomy with or without radiation and preoperative or postoperative chemotherapy can be performed. A marginal efficacy has been reported for the use of chemotherapy in localized resectable soft tissue sarcoma with respect to local recurrence, distant recurrence, overall recurrence, and overall survival.[12] Ablation procedures, embolization procedures, stereotactic body radiation therapy, or observation can also be considered.

G. For disseminated metastatic disease, palliation should be considered. Options include chemotherapy, radiation therapy, surgery, observation, supportive care, ablation procedures, or embolization procedures.

2. The excision site can be managed with tension-free primary approximation, skin graft, or flap; it is seldom healed by secondary intention.

3. For spermatic cord sarcoma, a radical inguinal orchiectomy with high ligation of the spermatic cord is recommended. Wide circumferential margins may be difficult to obtain because of anatomic constraints. Partial scrotectomy and resection of the surrounding tissues may be necessary. The major pattern of failure for spermatic cord sarcoma is local recurrence.

Combined surgery and radiation may be considered in patients who are at high risk (lesions >5 cm) for local failure.[13]

Basal cell carcinoma

1. Biopsy-proven lesions should be excised with 4-mm clinical margins. Mohs surgery can be performed alternatively.[14]

2. Margins should be assessed. If positive, surgical reexcision should be performed. If unable to obtain a negative margin, radiation therapy is recommended. If margins are negative but extensive perineural or large nerve involvement is present, radiation therapy is recommended.

3. No guidelines from the National Comprehensive Cancer Network are available for regional lymphadenopathy for basal cell carcinoma. Surgical management can be extrapolated from treatment of regional lymphadenopathy in squamous cell carcinoma. Fine needle aspiration or core biopsy should be performed for palpable regional lymph nodes or abnormal lymph nodes identified on imaging. If positive and operable, regional lymph node dissection should be performed. Radiation therapy should be considered if multiple lymph nodes are involved or if extracapsular extension is present. If regional lymph nodes are positive and inoperable, radiation therapy with or without systemic therapy is recommended.

4. The excision site can be managed with tension-free primary approximation, skin graft, or flap; it is seldom healed by secondary intention.

5. Nonsurgical candidates should receive radiation therapy.

6. Recent developments in systemic therapy, such as Hedgehog pathway inhibitor, may be an option for metastatic disease. Minimal evidence is available regarding chemotherapy.

Melanoma

1. Biopsy-proven lesions are treated according to stage. Scrotal melanoma management can be guided by the profusion of data on other skin melanoma sites, because no data specifically exist for scrotal-only melanomas.[15]

A. For stage 0 or IA and IB (<0.75 mm thick), wide excision should be performed based on tumor thickness.

B. For stage IA (0.76–1.00 mm thick), wide excision should be performed and consider sentinel lymph node biopsy. If sentinel lymph node biopsy is positive, see stage III.

C. For stage IB (0.76–1.00 mm thick) or stage II (>1.00 mm thick), wide excision should be performed and consider sentinel lymph node biopsy. If sentinel lymph node biopsy is positive, see stage III. If sentinel lymph node biopsy is negative, adjuvant therapy such as clinical trials, observation, or possibly interferon alfa can be considered.

D. For stage III (positive sentinel node), perform complete lymph node dissection. Adjuvant therapy clinical trials, observation, interferon alfa, or high-dose ipilimumab can be considered. Newer immunotherapy agents, including PD-1 inhibitors such as nivolumab and pembrolizumab, are currently being evaluated. They have preliminarily been shown to improve overall survival.[16]

E. For stage IV (metastatic disease) that is resectable, surgical resection should be performed. Systemic therapy can also be considered. For metastatic disease that is unresectable, options include systemic therapy, clinical trials, intralesional injection, or palliative resection with or without radiation therapy.

2. Excision site can be managed with tension-free primary approximation, skin graft, or flap and seldom, with healing by secondary intention (**Table 2**).

Adnexal tumors

1. Biopsy-proven lesions should be excised with a wide margin. Owing to the rarity of these tumors, adequate margins have not been evaluated in clinical trials or observational studies. In general, 1- to 2-cm clinical margins are recommended.[17]

2. No guidelines from the National Comprehensive Cancer Network are available for regional lymphadenopathy in adnexal tumors. However, because the staging of malignant cutaneous adnexal tumors is consolidated with the staging for cutaneous squamous cell carcinoma, surgical management of regional lymphadenopathy is likely similar. Fine needle aspiration or core biopsy should be performed for palpable

regional lymph nodes or abnormal lymph nodes identified on imaging. If positive and operable, regional lymph node dissection should be performed. Radiation therapy should be considered if multiple lymph nodes are involved or if extracapsular extension is present. If regional lymph nodes are positive and inoperable, radiation therapy with or without systemic therapy is recommended.

3. The excision site can be managed with tension-free primary approximation, skin graft, or flap and seldom, with healing by secondary intention.

4. Nonsurgical candidates should receive radiation therapy.

5. Minimal evidence is available regarding treatment of metastatic disease.

Case report

A 67-year-old Caucasian male presented with scrotal ulceration for 6 years. He had a previous scrotal exploration and incision and drainage 8 years prior for scrotal abscesses. He stated that the surgical incision dehisced and had never healed. The wound had worsened over time, constantly draining foul-smelling discharge. He reported a 25-pound weight loss over the past 6 months. His history was significant for an 80 pack-year smoking history. He did not report any chemical exposure, significant sun exposure, or other malignancies.

On examination, there is a 10-cm ulcerated condylomatous lesion involving the majority of his scrotum. The lesion spares the perineum and extends to the base of the ventral penis. Serous drainage is noted. The testes are palpable and involvement is unclear. There are palpable bilateral enlarged, freely mobile inguinal nodes.

Computed tomography scan of the chest, abdomen, and pelvis revealed enlarged bilateral external iliac chain lymph nodes, measuring up to 1.2 cm. There are also enlarged bilateral inguinal lymph nodes, measuring up to 1.8 cm. Nodular skin thickening and ulceration is noted involving the scrotum, which is abutting and inseparable from bilateral testicles. No hilar, mediastinal, retroperitoneal lymph nodes, or osseous lesions are reported.

Excisional biopsy of the lesion revealed invasive well-differentiated squamous cell carcinoma. The patient was consented for and taken to the operating room for cystoscopy, radical scrotectomy, bilateral simple orchiectomy, and reconstruction as a joint case with plastic surgery. Intraoperative photographs are presented (**Figs. 1–10**).

The patient had an uncomplicated postoperative course. Pathology revealed well-differentiated

Table 2		
Wide excision surgical margins for melanoma		
Tumor Thickness (mm)	**Recommended Clinical Margins (cm)**	
In situ	0.5–1.0	
≤1.00	1.0	
1.01–2.00	1.0–2.0	
2.01–4.00	2.0	
>4.00	2.0	

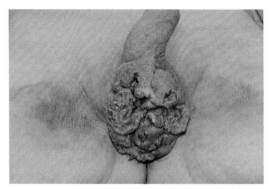

Fig. 1. The patient had a 10 cm ulcerating, condylomatous lesion on his scrotum. The penis and adjacent regions do not seem to be involved.

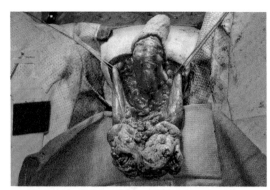

Fig. 4. The incision was carried through the skin, subcutaneous tissue, and dartos. The lesions seemed to involve the bilateral testes. The spermatic cords were isolated with vessel loops.

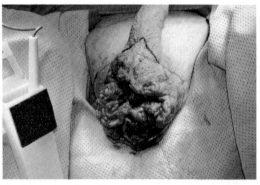

Fig. 2. He was placed in the exaggerated dorsal lithotomy position, widely prepped, and draped. The superior aspect of the lesion was circumferentially marked with clear clinical margins.

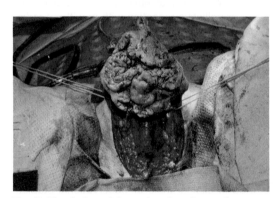

Fig. 5. The lesion did not involve the perineum or medial thighs.

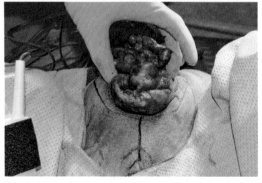

Fig. 3. The inferior aspect of the lesions was marked circumferentially with clear clinical margins.

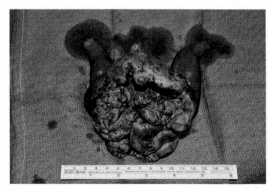

Fig. 6. The spermatic cords were ligated and the specimen was passed of the operating field.

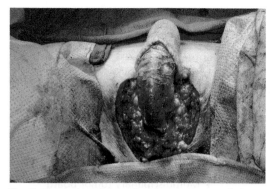

Fig. 7. The lesion did not involve the corporal tissues of the penis.

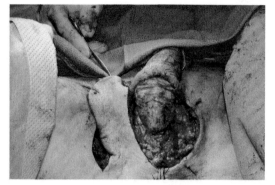

Fig. 8. A rotational skin and fascial flap was developed from the right medial thigh.

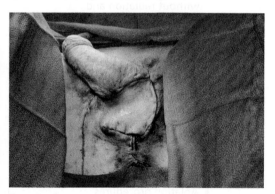

Fig. 9. The rotational flap provided adequate coverage for closure of the defect.

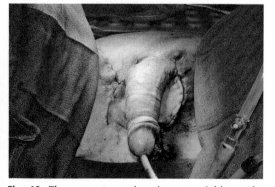

Fig. 10. The reconstructed region was viable at the end of the case.

Table 3
Complications and management

Complications	Management
Wound infection	• Antibiotics • May require opening the incision and drainage if abscess is present
Hematoma	• Resolution with time • Scrotal support • Drainage if infected
Pain	• Nonsteroidal anti-inflammatory drugs • Ice • Scrotal support

squamous cell carcinoma, extending to the deep dermal soft tissues. The testes were not involved. All margins were negative, with the closest margin measuring 0.3 cm. The patient was discussed at tumor board and the consensus was that no additional surgery, radiation, or chemotherapy was necessary. His follow-up PET scan was negative for residual or metastatic disease. His serial imaging has been negative and he is alive without evidence of disease (**Table 3**).

POSTOPERATIVE CARE

- Surgical removal of scrotal cancer can usually be performed as outpatient surgery.
- Nonsteroidal anti-inflammatory drugs, ice, scrotal support, and narcotics as needed are recommended for pain control and swelling.

Table 4
Stage and description

Stage	Description
A1	Localized to the scrotal wall
A2	Locally extensive tumor invading adjacent structure (testis, spermatic cord, penis, pubis, perineum)
B	Metastatic disease involving inguinal lymph node
C	Metastatic disease involving pelvic lymph nodes without evidence of distance spread
D	Metastatic disease beyond the pelvic lymph nodes involving distant organs

Adapted from Lowe FC. Squamous cell carcinoma of the scrotum. J Urol 1983;423–7; with permission.

Table 5
Follow-up time frame for evaluation and recurrence location and treatment

	Follow-up Time Frame and Evaluation	Recurrence Location and Treatment
Squamous cell carcinoma[9]	Local disease: • History and physical, including complete skin examination, every 3–12 mo for 2 y, then every 6–12 mo for 3 y, then annually for life • Patient education regarding sun protection and examination of skin Regional disease: • History and physical, including complete skin examination, every 1–3 mo for 1 y, then every 2–4 mo for 1 y, then every 4–6 mo for 3 y, then every 6–12 mo annually for life • Patient education regarding sun protection and examination of skin	Local: • Local excision New regional disease: • Regional lymph node dissection Regional recurrence or distant metastases: • Multidisciplinary tumor board consultation
Extramammary Paget's disease[10,19]	Close monitoring for long periods is recommended because recurrences are common because of subclinical disease; no recommended schedule is available	• Wide local excision • Adjuvant neodymium:YAG laser and topical 5-fluorouracil
Sarcoma[11]	Stage 1 disease: • History and physical, including complete skin examination, every 3–6 mo for 2–3 y, then annually for life • Chest imaging every 6–12 mo • Consider obtaining postoperative baseline and periodic imaging of primary site based on risk of locoregional recurrence • Evaluation for rehabilitation Stage II, III, and IV disease: • History and physical, including complete skin examination, and chest imaging every 3–6 mo for 2–3 y, then every 6 mo for 2 y, then annually for life • Consider obtaining postoperative baseline and periodic imaging of primary site based on risk of locoregional recurrence • Evaluation for rehabilitation	Local: • Local excision and treatment based on stage I, II, or III Isolated regional disease or nodes: • Regional node dissection with or without radiation and chemotherapy • Metastasectomy with or without radiation and preoperative or postoperative chemotherapy can be performed • Stereotactic body radiation therapy • Isolated limb perfusion Single organ and limited tumor bulk that is amenable to local therapy: • Metastasectomy with or without radiation and preoperative or postoperative chemotherapy can be performed • Ablation procedures • Embolization procedures • Stereotactic body radiation therapy Disseminated metastases: • Palliation, including chemotherapy, radiation therapy, surgery, observation, ablation procedures, embolization procedures
Basal cell carcinoma[14]	• History and physical, including complete skin examination, every 6–12 mo for life • Patient education regarding sun protection and examination of skin	Local: • Local excision Nodal or distant metastases: • Surgery and/or radiation therapy • Multidisciplinary tumor board consultation

(continued on next page)

Table 5
(continued)

	Follow-up Time Frame and Evaluation	Recurrence Location and Treatment
Melanoma[15]	Stage 0: • Annual complete skin examination for life • Education about regular self-skin and lymph node examination Stage IA-IIA NED: • History and physical, including complete skin examination, every 6–12 mo for 5 y, then annually as clinically indicated • Education about regular self -skin examination and lymph node examination • Routine radiologic imaging for asymptomatic recurrent/metastatic disease is not recommended Stage IIB-IV NED: • History and physical, including complete skin examination, every 3–6 mo for 2 y, then every 3–12 mo for 3 y, then annually as clinically indicated • Consider chest radiograph, CT, brain MRI, and/or PET/CT scans every 3–12 mo to screen for recurrent/metastatic disease • Routine radiologic imaging for asymptomatic recurrent/metastatic disease is not recommended after 3–5 y • Education about regular self-skin examination and lymph node examination	Persistent disease or local scar recurrence: • Reexcision to appropriate margins Local, satellite, and/or in-transit recurrence: • Clinical trial (preferred) • Local therapy, such as surgical excision, intralesional injection, ablation, topical imiquimod, radiation therapy • Regional therapy • Systemic therapy Nodal: • If no previous dissection, perform complete lymph node dissection and then adjuvant treatment • If previous dissection, perform complete lymph node dissection if possible and then adjuvant treatment • If unresectable, systemic therapy is preferred; can consider clinical trial, palliative radiation therapy, or intralesional injection Metastatic disease: • Follow treatment for stage IV (metastatic disease) melanoma
Adnexal skin tumors[17]	Routine follow-up is recommended as local recurrence rates range from 10%–50% among patients treated with wide local excision. No recommended schedule is available.	• Wide excision for local recurrence • Radiation therapy if surgical margins are positive • Metastatic disease is treated on a case by case basis

Abbreviations: CT, computed tomography; NED, no evidence of disease.

• Bacitracin ointment can be applied to surgical incision for 1 to 2 weeks.
• Showering is encouraged after 24 hours.
• Minimal exertion for 1 to 2 weeks.
• Postoperative follow-up in 1 to 2 weeks for evaluations and drain removal, if present.

REPORTING, FOLLOW-UP, AND CLINICAL IMPLICATIONS

The staging for scrotal cancer, reported by Lowe,[18] is shown in **Table 4**. However, because of the various histologic subtypes of scrotal cancer (ie, sarcoma and melanoma), many reports use the cancer staging system developed by the American Joint Committee on Cancer. Additionally, many reports do not provide sufficient information to determine staging (**Table 5**).

OUTCOMES

Because scrotal cancer is a rare disease and comprises multiple histologies, data regarding outcomes are limited. In an analysis of the Surveillance, Epidemiology, and End Results database for scrotal cancers, Johnson and colleagues[4] reported that the 6 histologic subtypes of scrotal cancers can be divided into 2 subgroups, with a higher and lower overall survival. Patients with basal cell carcinoma, extramammary Paget's

Table 6
SCC comorbidities, staging, surgical findings, and outcomes

	Comorbidities	Staging	Surgical Findings	Outcomes
Matoso et al,[20] 2014 (n = 29, median follow-up 37 mo)	Condylomas Other skin cancers Immunocompromised state (HIV, kidney transplantation) Leukemia/lymphoma Infection/inflammatory conditions Tanning bed use	In situ (19/29) Invasive (10/29) Inguinal lymphadenopathy (3/29)	Positive margins (13/29) Recurrence (3/29)	18 NED 3 alive with disease 3 deaths not from SCC 5 not available
Andrews et al,[6] 1991 (n = 14, mean follow-up 84 mo)	Psoriasis treated with coal tar and arsenic Human papillomavirus Cutaneous epitheliomas	Stage A1 (8/14) Stage B (3/14) Stage C (3/14)	Unknown	11 NED 3 deaths from SCC
Parys & Hutton,[21] 1991 (n = 11, median follow-up unknown)	Industrial exposure to machine oils and tar	Stage A1 (9/11) Stage B (1/11) Stage C (1/11)	Unknown	2 deaths from SCC 4 deaths not from SCC

Abbreviations: HIV, human immunodeficiency virus; NED, no evidence of disease; SCC, squamous cell carcinoma.

Table 7
Extramammary Paget's disease comorbidities, staging, surgical findings, and outcomes

	Comorbidities	Staging	Surgical Findings	Outcomes
Qi et al,[22] 2014 (n = 14, median follow-up 63 mo)	Other cancers	Lymph node metastasis (3/14) Distant metastasis (1/14)	Positive margins (5/14) Recurrence (1/14)	9 NED 2 alive with disease 2 deaths from EMPD 1 lost to follow-up
Park et al,[10] 2001 (n = 5, median follow-up 14 mo)	Unknown	Lymph node metastasis (1/5)	Unknown	5 NED
Chen et al,[23] 2013 (n = 30, mean follow-up 64.9 mo)	Unknown	Epidermis only (15/30) Epidermis with visceral or adnexal carcinoma (9/30) Lymph node metastasis (6/30)	Positive margins (2/30) Recurrence (8/30)	22 NED 5 deaths from EMPD
Zhang et al,[24] 2010 (n = 25, mean follow-up 119 mo)	Unknown	Stage A1 (10/25) Stage A2 (13/25) Stage B (1/25) Stage D (1/25)	Positive margins (5/25) Recurrence (7/25)	1 death from metastatic EMPD 6 deaths not from EMPD
Yang et al,[25] 2005 (n = 36, median follow-up 36 mo)	Unknown	Unknown	Positive margins (18/36) Recurrence (9/36)	1 death from metastatic EMPD
Koh et al,[26] 2015 (n = 5, median follow-up unknown)	Unknown	Dermis invasion (1/5) Dartos invasion (1/5) Inguinal lymph node metastasis (5/5) Pelvic lymph node metastasis (2/5) Distant metastasis (1/5)	Positive margins (1/5) Recurrence (3/5)	2 NED 3 alive with disease
Lai et al,[27] 2003 (n = 31, median follow-up unknown)	Unknown	Epidermis (14/31) Involving adnexal glands (10/31) Adnexal carcinoma (7/31)	Recurrence (6/31)	3 deaths from metastatic EMPD

Abbreviations: EMPD, extramammary paget's disease; NED, no evidence of disease.

Table 8
Sarcoma comorbidities, staging, surgical findings, and outcomes

	Comorbidities	Staging	Surgical Findings	Outcomes
Matoso et al,[28] 2014 (n = 5, median follow-up 6.5 mo)	Unknown	Infiltrative borders (0/5)	Positive margin (2/4, 1 not available) Recurrence (0/2, 3 not available)	2 NED 3 not available
Boland et al,[29] 2010 (n = 2, median follow-up 35 mo)	Unknown	Unknown	Unknown	2 NED
Froehner et al,[30] 2000 (n = 11, median follow-up 49 mo)	Unknown	Stage 1 (5/11) Stage 2 (4/11) Stage 3 (1/11) Stage 4 (1/11)	Recurrence (2/11)	10 NED 1 alive with disease
Ballo et al,[13] 2001 (n = 32, median follow-up 108 mo)	Unknown	T1 (≤5 cm) (15/32) T2 (>5 cm) (17/32)	Recurrence (12/32)	23 NED 9 deaths from sarcoma

Abbreviation: NED, no evidence of disease.

disease, and sarcoma were noted to have a higher overall survival, with median (95% CI) survival of 143 (116–180), 165 (139–190), and 180 (141–219) months, respectively. Patients with melanoma, squamous cell carcinoma, and adnexal tumors were noted to have a lower overall survival, with a median (95% CI) survival of 136 (70–203), 115 (97–133), and 114 (55–174) months, respectively. The 5-year overall survival for low-risk risk scrotal cancers (sarcoma, extramammary Paget's disease, basal cell carcinoma) and high-risk scrotal cancers (melanoma, squamous cell carcinoma, adnexal tumors) are about 75% and 55%, respectively. An extensive review of the literature was performed to assess outcomes from the various histologic subtypes of scrotal cancer. Outcomes from case series on squamous cell carcinoma, extramammary Paget's disease, sarcoma, basal cell carcinoma, and melanoma, based on histology, are provided in **Tables 6–10**. Outcomes from case reports were not included. No case series are available for adnexal tumors.

CURRENT CONTROVERSIES AND FUTURE CONSIDERATIONS

- Rare nature and small case series of scrotal cancers limits results regarding outcomes.
- Pooling of multiinstitutional data and the use of a scrotal cancer registry can improve knowledge of this disease and help develop treatment algorithms.

Table 9
Basal cell carcinoma comorbidities, staging, surgical findings, and outcomes

	Comorbidities	Staging	Surgical Findings	Outcomes
Dai et al,[31] 2012 (n = 10, mean follow-up 47 mo)	None	Reticular dermis (7/10) Subcutaneous tissue (1/10) Extending down to the Dartos muscle (2/10)	Positive margins (0/5) Recurrence (2/5)	8 NED

Abbreviation: NED, no evidence of disease.

Table 10
Melanoma comorbidities, staging, surgical findings, and outcomes

	Comorbidities	Staging	Surgical Findings	Outcomes
Sanchez-Ortiz et al,[32] 2005 (n = 6, median follow-up 39 mo)	Unknown	Inguinal metastasis (2/6)	Recurrence (3/6)	4 deaths from melanoma

SUMMARY

Primary scrotal cancer is a rare urologic malignancy. Pathologic assessment is necessary to determine the histologic subtype of this disease. The management for localized disease is surgical excision of the cancer with wide margins, because subclinical disease is often present. Lymph node metastases can also be managed with a regional lymph node dissection, although no trials have formally examined the usefulness of regional lymphadenectomy. Treatment for distant metastases is not as clear, with the use of various modalities in case reports.

Outcomes are also limited for this disease, with most data being reported in case series. Based on their analysis of the Surveillance, Epidemiology, and End Results database, Johnson and colleagues[4] noted that the 5-year overall survival for low-risk and high-risk scrotal cancers is about 75% and 55%, respectively. Interestingly, the 5-year relative survival for patients with penile cancer is reported to be 69%.[33] As such, high-risk scrotal cancers seem to have a worse prognosis and low-risk scrotal cancer may have comparable prognosis with penile cancer, a cutaneous urologic cancer in an adjacent region.

Occupational exposure to aromatic hydrocarbons is not as prevalent today, contributing to the decrease in scrotal cancers and limited data regarding this disease. Further work, including obtaining larger cohorts and the use of a database, can improve the management and information regarding long-term outcomes for scrotal cancer.

REFERENCES

1. Waldron HA. A brief history of scrotal cancer. Br J Ind Med 1983;40(4):390–401.
2. Melicow MM. Percivall Pott (1713-1788): 200th anniversary of first report of occupation-induced cancer scrotum in chimney sweepers (1775). Urology 1975; 6(6):745–9.
3. Azike JE. A review of the history, epidemiology and treatment of squamous cell carcinoma of the scrotum. Rare Tumors 2009;1(1):e17.
4. Johnson TV, Hsiao W, Delman KA, et al. Scrotal cancer survival is influenced by histology: a SEER study. World J Urol 2013;31(3):585–90.
5. Herrel LA, Weiss AD, Goodman M, et al. Extramammary Paget's disease in males: survival outcomes in 495 patients. Ann Surg Oncol 2015;22(5):1625–30.
6. Andrews PE, Farrow GM, Oesterling JE. Squamous cell carcinoma of the scrotum: long-term followup of 14 patients. J Urol 1991;146(5):1299–304.
7. Wolf JS Jr, Bennett CJ, Dmochowski RR, et al. Best practice policy statement on urologic surgery antimicrobial prophylaxis. J Urol 2008;179(4):1379–90.
8. Tanner J, Norrie P, Melen K. Preoperative hair removal to reduce surgical site infection. Cochrane Database Syst Rev 2011;(11):CD004122.
9. National Comprehensive Cancer Network (NCCN). NCCN clinical practice guidelines in oncology: squamous cell skin cancer. Fort Washington (PA): National Comprehensive Cancer Network; 2015.
10. Park S, Grossfeld GD, McAninch JW, et al. Extramammary Paget's disease of the penis and scrotum: excision, reconstruction and evaluation of occult malignancy. J Urol 2001;166(6):2112–6 [discussion: 2117].
11. National Comprehensive Cancer Network (NCCN). NCCN clinical practice guidelines in oncology: soft tissue sarcoma. Fort Washington (PA): National Comprehensive Cancer Network; 2016.
12. Pervaiz N, Colterjohn N, Farrokhyar F, et al. A systematic meta-analysis of randomized controlled trials of adjuvant chemotherapy for localized resectable soft-tissue sarcoma. Cancer 2008; 113(3):573–81.
13. Ballo MT, Zagars GK, Pisters PW, et al. Spermatic cord sarcoma: outcome, patterns of failure and management. J Urol 2001;166(4):1306–10.
14. National Comprehensive Cancer Network (NCCN). NCCN clinical practice guidelines in oncology: basal cell skin cancer. Fort Washington (PA): National Comprehensive Cancer Network; 2015.
15. National Comprehensive Cancer Network (NCCN). NCCN clinical practice guidelines in oncology: melanoma. Fort Washington (PA): National Comprehensive Cancer Network; 2015.
16. Long G, editor. Pembolizumab (pembro) + low-dose ipilimumab (ipi) for advanced melanoma. Society for

Melanoma Research 2015 Congress. San Francisco, November 18-21, 2015.

17. North JP, McCalmont TH, Ruben BS. Cutaneous adnexal tumors; 2015. Available at: http://www.uptodate.com/contents/cutaneous-adnexal-tumor.

18. Lowe FC. Squamous cell carcinoma of the scrotum. J Urol 1983;130(3):423–7.

19. Lopes Filho LL, Lopes IM, Lopes LR, et al. Mammary and extramammary Paget's disease. An Bras Dermatol 2015;90(2):225–31.

20. Matoso A, Ross HM, Chen S, et al. Squamous neoplasia of the scrotum: a series of 29 cases. Am J Surg Pathol 2014;38(7):973–81.

21. Parys BT, Hutton JL. Fifteen-year experience of carcinoma of the scrotum. Br J Urol 1991;68(4):414–7.

22. Qi Y, Hu J, Sun C, et al. Extramammary Paget's disease: analysis of 17 Chinese cases. Indian J Dermatol Venereol Leprol 2014;80(2):129–33.

23. Chen Q, Chen YB, Wang Z, et al. Penoscrotal extramammary Paget's disease: surgical techniques and follow-up experiences with thirty patients. Asian J Androl 2013;15(4):508–12.

24. Zhang N, Gong K, Zhang X, et al. Extramammary Paget's disease of scrotum–report of 25 cases and literature review. Urol Oncol 2010;28(1):28–33.

25. Yang WJ, Kim DS, Im YJ, et al. Extramammary Paget's disease of penis and scrotum. Urology 2005;65(5):972–5.

26. Koh YX, Tay TK, Xu S, et al. A clinical series and literature review of the management of inguinal nodal metastases in patients with primary extramammary Paget disease of the scrotum. Asian J Surg 2015;38(1):40–6.

27. Lai YL, Yang WG, Tsay PK, et al. Penoscrotal extramammary Paget's disease: a review of 33 cases in a 20-year experience. Plast Reconstr Surg 2003;112(4):1017–23.

28. Matoso A, Chen S, Plaza JA, et al. Symplastic leiomyomas of the scrotum: a comparative study to usual leiomyomas and leiomyosarcomas. Am J Surg Pathol 2014;38(10):1410–7.

29. Boland JM, Weiss SW, Oliveira AM, et al. Liposarcomas with mixed well-differentiated and pleomorphic features: a clinicopathologic study of 12 cases. Am J Surg Pathol 2010;34(6):837–43.

30. Froehner M, Lossnitzer A, Manseck A, et al. Favorable long-term outcome in adult genitourinary low-grade sarcoma. Urology 2000;56(3):373–7.

31. Dai B, Kong YY, Ye DW, et al. Basal cell carcinoma of the scrotum: clinicopathologic analysis of 10 cases. Dermatol Surg 2012;38(5):783–90.

32. Sanchez-Ortiz R, Huang SF, Tamboli P, et al. Melanoma of the penis, scrotum and male urethra: a 40-year single institution experience. J Urol 2005;173(6):1958–65.

33. Mosconi AM, Roila F, Gatta G, et al. Cancer of the penis. Crit Rev Oncol Hematol 2005;53(2):165–77.

Advances in Surgical Reconstructive Techniques in the Management of Penile, Urethral, and Scrotal Cancer

® CrossMark

Michael Bickell, DO, Jonathan Beilan, MD, Jared Wallen, MD,
Lucas Wiegand, MD, Rafael Carrion, MD*

KEYWORDS

• Penis • Urethra • Scrotum • Reconstruction • Cancer • Flap

KEY POINTS

- This article reviews the most up-to-date surgical treatment options for the reconstructive management of patients with penile, urethral, and scrotal cancer.
- Each organ system is examined individually, and the type of reconstructive surgical technique follows according to the primary oncologic procedure.
- Techniques and discussion for penile cancer reconstruction include Mohs surgery, glans resurfacing, partial and total glansectomy, and phalloplasty.
- Included in the penile cancer reconstruction section is the use of penile prosthesis in phalloplasty patients after penectomy, tissue engineering in phallic regeneration, and penile transplantation.
- Reconstruction following treatment of primary urethral carcinoma and current techniques for scrotal cancer reconstruction using split-thickness skin grafts and flaps are described.

The management of penile, urethral, and scrotal cancer consists of a myriad of treatment options that vary according to the type and severity of the oncologic pathology. The goal of reconstruction following surgical treatment of malignancy is to restore cosmesis, form, and function of the organ. For penile cancer, this entails retaining or restoring the ability to urinate while standing, achieve erection and sexual penetration, and maintaining erogenous sensation to the phallus or neo-phallus. The goal of reconstruction following treatment of urethral carcinoma is to recreate or reestablish normal voiding via anastomotic repair, urethral substitution, or urinary diversion. The primary goals of scrotal reconstruction consist of protecting the testes, epididymis, and cord structures and maintenance of an environment conducive to the production of spermatozoa and hormonal function.

In addition to the traditional techniques used in reconstructive urology, this article serves to highlight advances in this dynamic field treating the sequela of these complex malignancies. Each organ is discussed separately, and the reconstructive treatment options follow accordingly.

PENILE CANCER
Reconstruction of the Penis Based on Type and Extent of Penile Malignancy

Squamous cell carcinoma accounts for more than 95% of the cases of cancer of the penis, yet penile

Department of Urology, University of South Florida, Tampa, FL, USA
* Corresponding author. Department of Urology, University of South Florida, 2 Tampa General Circle, Mail Stop STC 6, Tampa, FL 33606.
E-mail address: rcarrion@health.usf.edu

Urol Clin N Am 43 (2016) 545–559
http://dx.doi.org/10.1016/j.ucl.2016.06.015
0094-0143/16/© 2016 Elsevier Inc. All rights reserved.

cancer remains an uncommon malignancy constituting less than 1% of all malignancies in men from developed countries.[1,2] The aim of treatment of penile cancer is to maximize organ preservation while achieving optimized oncologic outcomes. There are a multitude of surgical techniques and procedures to treat penile carcinoma that vary depending on the stage and grade of the penile malignancy.

Carcinoma In Situ, Ta, and T1 of the Penis

The first-line treatment option for carcinoma in situ (CIS) of the penis, erythroplasia of Queyrat, and Bowen disease is topical chemotherapy with imiquimod or 5-fluorouracil. In addition to topical agents, laser treatment, cryotherapy, circumcision, and photodynamic therapy may be used as alternative first-line treatment options.[3] There are no randomized studies comparing organ-preserving and ablative treatment strategies from an oncologic standpoint, only retrospective studies with level 3 evidence or less; as ablative therapies require less reconstruction postoperatively given their inherent nature, the authors omit discussion of reconstruction following ablative procedures. Total or partial glans resurfacing as well as Mohs surgery may be offered as both a primary treatment option or as a secondary-line treatment of CIS and noninvasive disease that is refractory to topical or laser therapy. A discussion on glans resurfacing and Mohs surgery follows. Local recurrence of penile Tis, Ta, and T1 tumors has little influence on long-term survival, thereby justifying organ preservation whenever possible for these lesions.[4–7]

Glans Resurfacing

The most common presenting location for malignant penile cancer is found on the glans and/or prepuce, with approximately 78% of the lesions detected at this location.[8] Glans resurfacing is one of the few techniques used to treat noninvasive penile cancer that is confined to the glans. It is important to note, however, that up to 20% of patients initially diagnosed with noninvasive penile cancer will have invasive disease at final pathology.[9] In one contemporary study of glans resurfacing, approximately 28% of patients treated with glans resurfacing required additional surgery for understaging of their disease or positive surgical margins at final pathology; however, the additional surgery was found not to compromise oncologic control.[9]

Total glans resurfacing is performed by first marking the glans epithelium in 4 quadrants starting at the meatus and extending to the coronal sulcus in each quadrant. Next a perimeatal incision is made followed by a circumferential coronal incision in each quadrant; the epithelial tissue is then completely excised off the spongiosum in each quadrant allowing for a completely exposed glans. Next deep biopsies are taken from the spongiosal tissue in each quadrant. Following biopsies a split-thickness skin graft (STSG) is used to cover the glans (**Fig. 1**).

Sexual function following glans resurfacing sheds light on the importance of this procedure and helps to serve as a reminder of the value of cancer survivorship objectives. In one study consisting of 10 patients who had undergone glans resurfacing for the treatment of erythroplasia of Queyrat, sexual function was evaluated at 6 months postoperatively.[10] All patients who were sexually active preoperatively remained sexually active at 6 months postoperatively. In this specific study, all patients denied a negative change in the sensation of the tip of the penis or a negative change in their sex life.

STSG is a common technique adapted from plastic surgery and used by urologists commonly for reconstructive purposes covering major skin loss while providing satisfactory functional and cosmetic outcomes. STSG is highlighted throughout this article, as it has many applications in reconstruction of the phallus and scrotum following surgical treatment of these malignancies. It is important to note that advanced reconstructive techniques including STSG demand that medical comorbidities be optimized before surgical intervention. This requirement is especially true for smokers; current evidence from the plastic surgery literature suggest that a period of cessation no less than 2 to 4 weeks before surgery should be followed to optimize outcomes and wound healing.[11]

Mohs Surgery for Carcinoma In Situ, Ta, and T1

Dr Frederic E. Mohs developed the surgical technique that bears his name in the 1930s while working on research as a medical student at the University of Wisconsin.[12] Mohs micrographic surgery (MMS) is a technique that involves excision of tissue in layers with microscopic examination of the undersurface of the tissue to ensure a clear margin of resection. MMS allows for maximal tissue preservation by using microscopically ensured oncologic resection. MMS has been used in the treatment of penile cancer for more than 50 years.[13] There have been several long-term studies that have evaluated the efficacy of MMS for penile carcinoma in terms of oncologic control

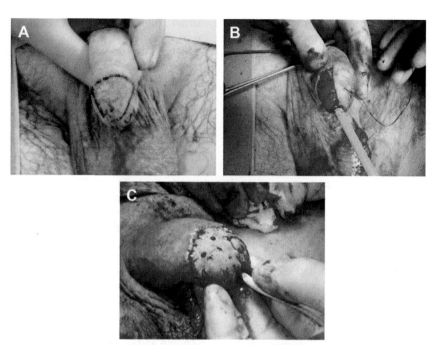

Fig. 1. (*A*) The glans epithelium is marked in quadrants from the meatus to the coronal sulcus; (*B*) glans epithelium and subepithelial tissue completely dissected off the underlying spongiosum, starting from the meatus to the coronal sulcus for each quadrant; (*C*) a STSG is sutured and quilted using multiple 5-0 interrupted sutures. (*From* Shabbir M, Muneer A, Kalsi J, et al. Glans resurfacing for the treatment of carcinoma in situ of the penis: surical technique and outcomes. Eur Urol 2011;59(1):144; with permission.)

and cosmetic outcomes. Brown and colleagues[14] studied 20 patients with both penile CIS and invasive disease and followed these patients for an average of 3 years. They reported a 29% recurrence rate during that follow-up period, with one patient ultimately dying of metastatic disease and 4 patients developing lymph node involvement. In a more contemporary study with a longer follow-up of almost 5 years, Shindel and colleagues[7] performed MMS on 41 penile cancers with a 32% recurrence rate. In total 25 of the cancers were CIS, 10 were invasive SCC, and 4 were Ta. Despite a high recurrence rate in patients treated with MMS compared with traditional surgery, the recurrence was effectively retreated and did not have an adverse effect on overall survival or tumor progression. It is important to note that only 13 of the defects created by MMS were amenable to primary closure; the remaining defects required skin grafts or tissue flaps. Overall MMS offers an excellent option in appropriately selected patients in minimizing sexual and urinary dysfunction postoperatively while achieving oncologic control. These patients must be agreeable, however, to vigilant long-term postoperative surveillance. Overall MMS allows for precise surgical approach, technique, and excision with a postsurgical bed that is microscopically free from tumor or

dysplastic changes; but based on the surprisingly high rate of recurrence, this treatment approach has fallen out of favor now.

Treatment of invasive disease confined to the corpus spongiosum and glans includes total glansectomy with or without resurfacing of the corporeal heads; partial amputation is considered for patients who are unfit for reconstruction.[3] Treatment of disease invading the corpora cavernosa or urethra (T2/T3) includes partial amputation with a tumor-free margin with reconstruction.

The armamentarium for the urologist in treating penile cancers in patients with T1, T2, or T3 disease includes total or partial glansectomy with reconstruction, wide local excision or partial penectomy with reconstruction, or total penectomy. Important considerations to best evaluate surgical outcomes include oncologic control, sexual function, cosmesis, psychosocial impact, and ability to void. Given these parameters, organ-sparing techniques and genital reconstruction have become paramount for patient satisfaction. A surgical margin of 5 mm is considered safe, but patients should remain under close follow-up.[15,16]

Partial glansectomy can include wide local excision of any of the glandular tissue and includes glans resurfacing, MMS, and true partial glansectomy. Total glansectomy includes making a subcoronal incision with removal of all the glandular tissue distal to the corona while preserving the entire length of the mature corporal cavernosal tissue. Some smaller lesions treated with partial glansectomy may be amenable to primary closure; however, multiple reconstructive techniques exist including local flaps or free grafts. There exists considerable overlap in the usage of flap or grafting techniques regardless of primary excision technique (partial glansectomy, total glansectomy, or partial penectomy). Local flaps include rotational flaps from preputial skin, scrotal skin, or urethral tissue. In a recent study published by Yang and colleagues,[17] 105 patients underwent glans-sparing excision of penile tumors less than 2.5 cm in diameter with either primary repair or preputial skin flap reconstruction. Skin flap reconstruction patients showed better 5-point satisfaction scale ratings in respect to orgasmic function, intercourse satisfaction, and overall satisfaction compared with primary repair patients at the 6-month follow-up. Free grafts include both buccal mucosa and STSG. However, Palminteri and colleagues[18] suggest that the nonnative environment of buccal mucosa to an external recipient site of the glans penis or distal shaft make it an inferior choice in this situation and prefer STSG.

Partial penectomy includes removal of any penile tissue en bloc distal to a circumferential line of demarcation that preserves a negative margin. After deep frozen sections have been taken to ensure a negative margin, the corporal bodies are closed with a 2-0 absorbable suture. The corpora spongiosum and urethra are spatulated ventrally and a neo-meatus is created. Classic thinking suggests that a 3-cm stump should be the minimal length left to preserve the ability to void from a standing position and negate the need for a total penectomy with perineal urethrostomy. The current guidelines from the National Comprehensive Cancer Network state that, for high-grade T1 and T2 or greater tumors, more invasive approaches, such as partial or total penectomy, are warranted; however, in a highly motivated and reliable patient, glansectomy with negative tumor margin is acceptable if close follow-up is ensured.[19] Again glanuloplasty can be performed with any of the aforementioned reconstructive techniques; however, Belinky and colleagues[20] in the *Journal of Urology* describes 10 patients treated with partial penectomy and urethral flap glanuloplasty with good cosmetic outcome and no incidence of meatal stenosis. After standardized partial penectomy with prior release of the pendulous urethra from the specimen, the urethra is spatulated ventrally to the level of the neo-meatus and then sutured to the distal ends of the corporal bodies as a flap glanuloplasty (**Fig. 2**).

The importance of psychosocial and sexual outcomes for patients after glansectomy or partial penectomy cannot be overstated. A recent study

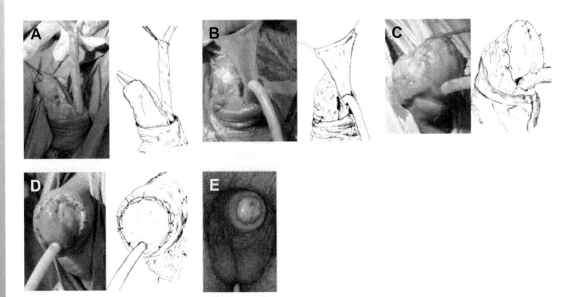

Fig. 2. (*A*) Urethral release up to penoscrotal junction; (*B*) urethral ventral spatulation; (*C*) urethral suture to distal end of cavernous bodies; (*D*) final outcome; (*E*) 6 months postoperatively. (*From* Belinky JJ, Cheliz GM, Graziano CA, et al. Glanuloplasty with urethral flap after partial penectomy. J Urol 2011;185(1):205; with permission.)

by Gulino and colleagues[21] documented good sexual outcomes with glansectomy and limited partial penectomy. In fact, 73%, 76%, and 71% of their 42 patients had rigid erections, retained normal orgasm and ejaculation, and preserved libido, respectively, at 6 months' follow-up after surgery. Although good outcomes are attainable with primary excision and the reconstructive techniques mentioned earlier, adjunctive reconstructive techniques can and should be used to further enhance quality of life and limit the psychosocial impact of intervention. These techniques include suspensory ligament release, ventral phalloplasty, and suprapubic lipectomy. In a recent video published in the *International Brazilian Journal of Urology*, Wallen and colleagues[22] document combined partial penectomy with ventral phalloplasty to preserve penile length. The video shows partial penectomy of an approximate 4-cm tumor with loss of only 2.5 cm of functional penile length after ventral phalloplasty (**Fig. 3**). Suprapubic lipectomy and suspensory ligament release have long been used as adjuncts in cosmetic urology and have a role in post–partial penectomy patients as well.

Reconstructive Options Following Total Penectomy

In the treatment of disease that is locally advanced invading adjacent structures (T3/T4), total penectomy with perineal urethrostomy is the standard surgical treatment of T3 tumors.[16] In more advanced T4 disease, neoadjuvant chemotherapy is advisable.

The standard of care for the treatment of advanced penile carcinoma T3 and T4 disease is a total penectomy with perineal urethrostomy often times accompanied or preceded by chemotherapy, particularly for T4 disease.[3,16] The

psychological effects of subtotal or total penectomy are often devastating on the quality of life of surviving patients as radical penile surgery affects sexual, voiding, and psychological well-being. Total phallic reconstruction was driven in part by the need in cancer survivors but also by trauma patients, disorders of sexual development, congenital anomalies, and female-to-male transsexual surgery. Perhaps no other need has greater advanced this field then genitoperineal transformation surgery in female-to-male transsexuals.

The origins of phallic reconstruction, however, were borne out of necessity on trauma patients with the first reported phalloplasty performed in 1936 by Russian surgeon Nikolaj Bogoraz.[23] Bogoraz's phalloplasty operation consisted of several stages, which began with the formation of bilateral tube pedicled grafts of the abdominal skin, then incorporated an 8-cm long segment of rib cartilage as a stiffner into the graft, and in a later stage reconstructed a portion of the urethra using a tubular scrotal flap. There were several surgical innovators that advanced the technique Bogoraz popularized, including Frumkin, Maltz, Gillies, and Harrison, by incorporating the tube within a tube concept of neo-urethral formation.[24] It was the advent of microsurgical techniques that truly ushered in a new era of penile reconstruction lead by Dr Song and further popularized by Chang and Hwang with the use of the radial artery free flap, which has become the most common technique used today and is universally considered the standard technique for total phallic reconstruction.[24] Since the introduction of microsurgical techniques and advancements in composite flaps, there has been a multitude of different approaches for total phallic reconstruction with more than 20 different types of flaps available.[25] It is beyond the scope of the article to review each type of flap, free or pedicled; but instead the authors

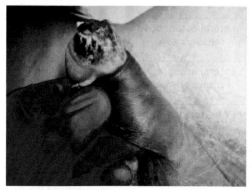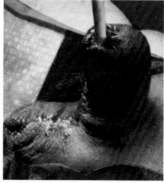

Fig. 3. Before and after images of partial penectomy patient with ventral phalloplasty performed at time of partial penectomy to maximize functional penile length.

review the most common flaps and advancements in these techniques as they pertain to reconstruction following penectomy for cancer.

There are many types of both pedicled and free soft tissue flaps used for penile reconstruction. The most common types of flaps used are listed later. This list is not exhaustive but shows the number and type of the more common flaps used today. Local pedicled flaps for phalloplasty included extended groin skin flaps, rectus abdominis myocutaneous flap, the superficial inferior epigastric skin flap, anterolateral thigh flap, and the tensor fascia lata myocutaneous flap. Soft tissue flaps include radial forearm flap, dorsalis pedis flap, deltoid flap, lateral arm flap, fibular flap, tensor fascia lata flap, latissimus dorsi flap, radial forearm osteocutaneous free flaps, and scapular flaps (**Table 1**).

The goals of free flap phalloplasty should include a one-stage procedure, creation of a competent genitoperineal that allows patients to void while standing, restoration of erogenous and tactile sensation, a neo-phallus that allows for insertion of a prosthetic device or alternative to allow for sexual function, an aesthetic and cosmetically acceptable result in both the donor and graft site, and minimizing scarring and disfigurement with no loss of function of the donor site.[26]

Radial Artery Free Flap Phalloplasty

Radial artery free flap (RAFF) is by far the most common flap used in total phallic reconstruction, with greater than 90% of reported cases using this technique. In a brief summary of the procedure described by Monstrey and colleagues,[27] the plastic surgeon first dissects the radial forearm flap and constructs a tube within a tube phallus. The glans is then sculpted with a small skin flap and a full-thickness skin graft while the neo-phallus is still attached to the forearm by its vascular pedicle. The urethra stump is then prepared; and the receptor vessels are then dissected in the groin, often through a lower abdominal incision; and the RAFF is transferred from the forearm to the pubic area. The urethral anastomosis is performed first, then the radial artery is anastomosed microscopically in an end-to-side fashion to the common

Table 1
Free and local pedicled flaps for phalloplasty

Type of Flap	Tissue Used	Innervation	Blood Supply	Pedicle Length
Groin flap	Skin & fat	Not sensate	Superficial circumflex iliac artery	2–5 cm
Rectus flap	Skin, fat, fascia, & muscle	Intercostal nerves	Deep inferior epigastric artery and vein	5–7 cm
Superficial inferior epigastric skin flap	Skin & fat	Not sensate	Superficial inferior epigastric artery and vein	3–5 cm
Anterolateral thigh flap	Skin, fat, & fascia	Lateral femoral cutaneous nerve	Descending branch of the lateral femoral circumflex artery	7 cm+
Tensor fascia lata flap	Skin, fascia, & muscle	Lateral cutaneous sensory nerve	Ascending branch of the lateral femoral circumflex artery	10 cm
Radial forearm free flap	Skin & fascia with tendon and bone as optional	Lateral antebrachial cutaneous nerve	Radial artery	Free flap
Lateral arm free flap	Skin, fat, & fascia; bone as optional	Posterior cutaneous nerve of forearm	Posterior radial collateral artery	Free flap
Fibula free flap	Skin, fat, & bone	Not sensate	Peroneal artery	Free flap
Latissimus flap	Skin & muscle	Thoracodorsal nerve	Thoracodorsal artery	10–15 cm
Scapular flap	Skin & fat	Not sensate	Transverse branch of circumflex scapular artery	3–7 cm

femoral artery, and the cephalic vein is anastomosed to the saphenous vein. An antebrachial nerve is microscopically anastomosed to the ipsilateral ilioinguinal nerve to allow for protective sensation, and another forearm nerve is connected to the dorsal nerve of the penis or pudendal nerves to allow for erogenous sensation[27,28] (Fig. 4).

Despite the RAFF as the most common technique used for phalloplasty, there is a paucity of prospective randomized controlled trials comparing flap techniques; therefore, it is not possible to prove one technique's superiority over another.[27] However, the RAFF has the most

long-term data and largest data series to date in total phallic reconstruction and has proven to be a reliable technique. The RAFF has the theoretic advantage of maintaining the greatest degree of sensitivity to the phallus both in tactile sensation as well as erogenous sensation based on previous studies examining radial forearm flaps in oral reconstruction.[29] Sensation of the RAFF phalloplasty is maintained via microsurgical anastomosis of the antebrachial nerves to the dorsal nerve of the penis or iliohypogastric and ilioinguinal nerves.

There are several drawbacks to the RAFF, the most common being donor site morbidity and

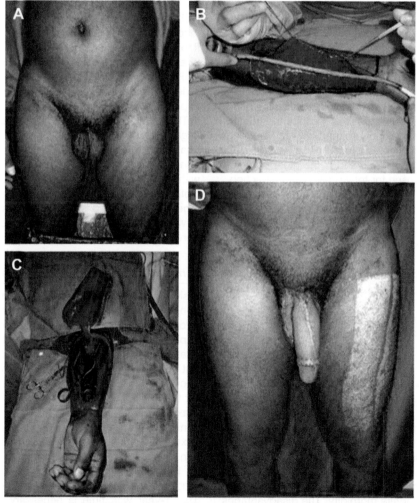

Fig. 4. (A) Preoperative view of a 38-year-old man following total penectomy and bilateral inguinal node dissection for invasive squamous cell cancer 8 months previously. The patient has perineal urethra. (B) Left radial forearm osteocutaneous flap prelamination of neo-urethra. (C) Radial forearm osteocutaneous flap shown following flap harvest before pedicle division and transfer. (D) The patient at 4 months following total phalloplasty with radial forearm osteocutaneous flap and adjunctive palmaris longus tendon graft for coronoplasty. (*From* Salgado CJ, Monstrey S, Hoebeke P, et al. Reconstruction of the penis after surgery. Urol Clin North Am 2010;37(3): 396; with permission.)

the need for a secondary operation to allow for implantation of a penile prosthesis to restore sexual function. The RAFF used in phalloplasty surgery is typically larger than what is commonly used in head and neck reconstruction, thus there is greater concern for functional impairment and a cosmetically undesirable result of the donor site. However, in a long-term follow-up study of sex reassignment patients, there were few major long-term problems identified at the donor site, including no functional limitation, chronic pain, or cold intolerance.[30] One of the most dreaded complications of any free flap phalloplasty is acute venous thrombosis of the anastomosis, which occurs with an incidence of 3%. Another dreaded vascular complication is acute thrombosis of the arterial anastomosis, which occurs soon after the anastomosis and is typically easily identifiable allowing for re-exploration and immediate revision and salvage of the phallus. The most common urologic complication of RAFF phalloplasty is urethral strictures and fistulas. Neo-urethral strictures, including meatal stenosis, occur in approximately 10% of the cases, whereas urethral fistulas occur in as many as 20% of cases. Despite the complication rates and donor site morbidity and scarring, the RAFF phalloplasty remains a reliable and reproducible technique and is the most common technique chosen for total phallic reconstruction.

Additional Flap Techniques

As previously stated, there are currently more than 20 techniques used in phallic reconstruction; the purpose of this article is not to review all of them but to highlight the most common and comment on the advancements in penile reconstruction. With this in mind, there have been recent flaps and advancements that deserve mention, namely, the osteocutaneous free flaps and the latissimus dorsi flap.

Radial and Fibular Osteocutaneous Free Flaps

These techniques were first described in 1993 with the inherent advantage of intrinsic rigidity of the flap allowing for sexual activity without the need for a prosthesis. The fibula free flap provides vascularized bone that is longer than the radial forearm osteocutaneous flap, thereby optimizing sexual outcomes; it is typically associated with reduced donor site morbidity. The disadvantages of the osteocutaneous flaps include a higher rate of urethral complications, including fistula and stricture; a permanently erect phallus; and less erogenous and tactile sensation of the neo-phallus.[28] The largest follow-up study for male patients treated with an osteocutaneous free fibular

flap phalloplasty includes 18 patients with an average follow-up of 5.5 years. The results of the follow-up study show no significant osseous resorption; good functional results, both urinary and sexual; and high patient satisfaction.[31] Long-term follow-up studies for radial forearm osteocutaneous flaps have shown softening of the neo-phallus, with approximately 20% of the patients seeking a corrective procedure at a mean of 2 years postoperatively[32]; refer to **Fig. 4** for surgical images of a radial forearm osteocutaneous flap.

Total phallic reconstruction using a musculocutaneous latissimus dorsi (MLD) flap was first described by Perovic and colleagues[33] in 2006 used in children as an alternative to the RAFF.[34] The group later published their results with this technique on adults necessitating total phallic reconstruction with the intention of providing a flap that allowed for creation of a larger neo-phallus with lower donor site morbidity then the RAFF. The MLD phalloplasty requires 4 stages in order to provide a functional neo-phallus that is capable to use for intercourse.

The advantages of the MLD are related to the larger size graft resulting in creation of a larger phallus and the limited donor site morbidity. The donor site can be closed directly in most patients without the need for additional tissue grafting, and clothing generally conceals its site. The disadvantage of the MLD flap is that it requires 4 stages, 2 of which require urethroplasty with buccal mucosa harvest as part of stage one of the urethroplasty.

Penile Prosthesis in Phalloplasty Patients

A significant advancement in phalloplasty patients concerns the insertion of a penile prosthesis in an effort to restore sexual function. Penile prosthesis implantation in phalloplasty patients remains a challenging procedure for the implant urologist but has long-term data proving its safety and efficacy. The prosthesis is inserted at least 1 year after the phallic reconstruction in order to allow for maximal nerve sensation, including cutaneous sensation, to develop. Previous studies on transsexual patients have shown that by 1 year, genital sensitivity and tactile sensitivity was regained[35]; to the authors' knowledge there are no such studies that exist on postpenectomy patients. This 1-year wait time is necessary to allow for sensation of the phallus to ensure both the erogenous enjoyment of the prosthesis as well as to ensure somatic sensation to help maintain the safety of the phallus in the event of extrusion or erosion. Both semirigid penile implants as well as inflatable penile implants have been used in the neo-phallus; both single cylinders as well as bilateral cylinders have been used.

The technique described by Zuckerman and colleagues[36] for insertion of a penile prosthesis in a neo-phallus begins with bilateral incisions overlying the ischial tuberosities (**Fig. 5**). In postpenectomy patients in which the proximal corpora remain, the standard technique is to open the proximal corpora and use them as the anchoring site of the prosthesis; this approach can be either penoscrotal or via bilateral incisions over the ischial tuberosities. Alternatively if the proximal corpora have been excised, the inferior pubic rami can be exposed and used as sites to anchor the prosthesis. The neo-phallus shaft is dilated distally in the standard fashion as with a typical implant with Metzenbaum scissors, Hager sounds, Brooks dilators, or a combination thereof. After appropriate sizing with the Furlow device, the implant is chosen and encased in polyethylene terephthalate creating a neo-tunica. The neo-tunica covering allows not only fixation of the cylinders to the proximal corpora or inferior pubic

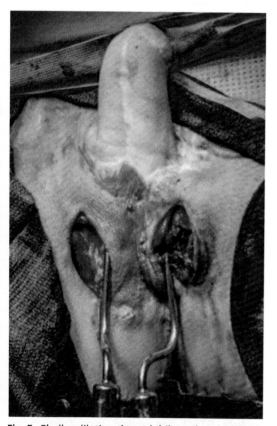

Fig. 5. Phallus dilation through bilateral perineal incisions. (*From* Zuckerman JM, Smentkowski K, Gilbert D, et al. Penile prosthesis implantation in patients with a history of total phallic construction. J Sex Med 2015;12(12):2487; with permission.)

rami but also protects against extrusion of the device through the glans of the neo-phallus by creating an added buffer between the implant and the skin. The cylinders are then placed in a standard fashion with the aid of a Keith needle and Furlow passer if an inflatable penile prosthesis is chosen, otherwise standard implantation of a semirigid implant commences at this point. After seating of the implant, the proximal end of the neo-tunica is sutured to the proximal corpora or inferior pubic ramus. If an inflatable device is chosen, the pump and reservoir need to be placed. The pump is placed in the scrotum through one of the perineal incisions after blunt creation of a subdartos pouch. The reservoir is placed via a lower abdominal counterincision.

As with any penile implant surgery infection, erosion into the urethra, extrusion from the skin, and mechanical failure are all possible complications of either type of implant, semirigid or inflatable. A recent study of penile implants in patients with a neo-phallus demonstrated a 6% intraoperative complication rate, including a cystotomy and a vascular flap injury. The postoperative revision rate was 23.0%, with a 9.7% infection rate. At 5 years' follow-up, approximately 80% of the patients were sexually active.[36] The largest series of penile implants in patients with a neo-phallus demonstrated a slightly higher infection rate of 12% and noted a significantly higher incidence of 41% for removal and revision.[37] Both studies used semirigid implants as well as inflatable implants but moved to preferring inflatable implants as the surgeons gained experience in placing penile implants in a neo-phallus. It is important to note that in the largest study only female-to-male transsexuals were included.

Tissue Engineering in Phallic Regeneration

Regenerative medicine is the process of replacing or regenerating human cells, tissues, or organs with the goal of restoration of structure and function.[38] There are in essence 3 different conceptual approaches for tissue engineering: autologous or allogeneic stem cells obtained from a biopsy and expanded in vitro, implantation of biological materials to assist tissue repair, and implantation of matrices that are seeded with stem cells.[39] Several trials have shown the potential of tissue-engineered corpus cavernosum as an alternative for surgical total phallic reconstruction.[40,41] Based on these studies, entire corporal bodies have been created using acellular corporal matrices seeded with autologous smooth muscle and endothelial cells in animals.[42] These studies have led to bioengineered corpora allowing male rabbits to successfully mate with female rabbits. Although predominately the studies have been conducted in animals, there are studies of human corpus cavernosal, endothelial, and smooth muscle cells, which have formed vascularized corporal bodies when implanted in vivo ex situ.[41]

Despite the dramatic advancements being made in tissue engineering, the promise of phallic reconstruction using stem cells does not as of yet have clinical utility in humans but remains a promising technology in the future.

Penile Transplantation

There are only 2 reports of penile transplantation in the medical literature. The first reported penile transplant was in 2006 in Guangzhou, China. The recipient was a 44-year-old man that suffered a traumatic event resulting in penile amputation. Following the appropriate medical and psychological workup, the 15-hour surgery was performed. The recipient was able to urinate after Foley catheter removal on postoperative day number 10 and showed no signs of rejection or infection. Unfortunately, because of extreme psychological distress of the patient and his wife, he requested the transplanted penis to be removed.[43] The second reported case of a penile transplant was performed in South Africa in 2014 following a traumatic amputation. The 21-year-old recipient underwent a 9-hour procedure and has recovered successfully with restoration of both urinary and sexual function.[44]

Both of these cases highlight the feasibility and success of a penile transplant, but more research is currently being investigated in an effort to improve outcomes for recipients. In both cases of penile transplantation, only the dorsal arteries, nerves, and veins were microscopically anastomosed. The cavernosal arteries and the bulbourethral arteries were not reapproximated directly. The cavernosal arteries are responsible for erection, but it is technically difficult to perform this anastomosis, as it requires excision and shortening of the native corpora in order to visualize the vessels and perform the anastomosis. Surgeons at Johns Hopkins University have investigated this issue and have shown that it is possible to revascularize a penile transplant with anastomosis of the dorsal, cavernosal, and external pudendal arteries in cadaveric trials that were complete with perfusion studies after anastomosis.[45] The cavernosal artery anastomosis was accomplished by gaining additional length of the donor penile allograft cavernosal arteries allowing for an anastomosis and less excision of recipient corporal tissue to expose the vessels. In addition to the cavernosal arteries, the external pudendal arteries were anastomosed via a groin incision to allow for improved perfusion of the penile shaft skin. The perfusion studies showed that corporal inflow was significantly improved compared with studies with solely dorsal artery anastomosis, suggesting improved results of erectile function with cavernosal artery anastomosis. No attempts were made during these studies to perform a bulbourethral anastomosis because of the size and shorter course of these arteries. Penile transplant offers an exciting alternative to flap phalloplasty and will likely be implemented in the next 12 months in the United States, mainly for patients with postwar traumatic amputation; however, this technique can be used in postpenectomy patients for malignancy as well. At the time of this article submission, Johns Hopkins School of Medicine was the only center in the United States that formalized a penile transplant program and was actively awaiting their first patient.

SCROTAL CANCER RECONSTRUCTION

Scrotal carcinoma as either primary malignancy or as extension from contiguous malignancy is a rare event; Surveillance, Epidemiology, and End Results' data estimate an age-adjusted incidence rate of 10 cases per 10 million persons of primary scrotal carcinoma.[46] Reconstruction of the scrotum and perineal area frequently requires the combined expertise of both urologic and plastic surgery teams. Tissue loss may be secondary to a variety of pathologies ranging from cancer to trauma and infection. A common cause for significant loss of scrotal tissue is surgical debridement of Fournier gangrene. Thus, most of the scientific literature regarding scrotal reconstruction involves this disease process and the techniques used to rebuild the scrotal and perineal architecture destroyed by Fournier's debridement. These reconstructive strategies are pertinent in the discussion of urologic oncology, as the resection of part or all of the scrotum may occur during patients' oncologic management.

The primary objectives in the reconstruction of scrotal and perineal wounds are to protect the testes (should they remain) and to close the defect in a secure and cosmetic fashion. Although the characteristic vascularity and redundancy of the scrotum allow for primary closure of a defect with skin loss up to 50%,[47] often the defect requires more involved efforts. Subcutaneous thigh pockets, STSG, and several myocutaneous and fasciocutaneous flaps have been used to achieve these goals.

Primary closure of the scrotum and perineal area is recommended whenever surgically sound. The final closure should not only protect the gonads but also provide good abutment of tissues in an effort to deliver tension-free healing. When simple primary closure is not feasible, the surgeon may explore other options, such as tissue-expanding techniques. Tissue-expanding musculocutaneous flaps constructed from the remnant scrotum have been shown to successfully close wounds with up to 67% skin loss of the scrotum.[48] Nevertheless, such efforts may be insufficient with very large surgical defects and associated tissue loss.

Often, delayed reconstruction of the scrotum is necessary because of ongoing infection, the need for further surgical debridement, or anesthesia risks. While awaiting definitive reconstruction, the denuded testicles may either be managed with regular wet dressing changes or buried within ipsilateral, medial, subcutaneous thigh pouches.[28] It has been well-established that, although thigh pouches offer a more expeditious repair with fewer postoperative wound complications, patients may ultimately have psychological dissatisfaction due to an absent scrotum as well as chronic pain at the implanted site as a result of repetitive mechanical trauma.[49] Furthermore, consideration must be given to the patients' age and fertility status. The scientific literature is sparse with regard to the effect various scrotal reconstruction techniques have on long-term testicular function and spermatogenesis. Demir and colleagues[50] demonstrated scrotal reconstruction using skin flaps, as opposed to skin grafts, that resulted in superior spermatogenesis in rat models at 2 months after the procedure. Other small case series have demonstrated that the scrotum's role as the testicles' thermoregulator is disrupted when the testes are covered with thick skin flaps or buried within thigh pouches.[51] This spermatogenesis arrest may be inhibited by thin-trimming the reconstruction flap at a later date[52]; however, this strategy has not been widely reproduced in the literature. Although controversy surrounds the best method of management, it is generally accepted that should patients desire to remain fertile, creation of a neo-scrotum or skin graft reconstruction is optimal because of the decreased rates of spermatogenesis associated with thigh pouches.

Meshed STSGs have several innate advantages as coverage of the exposed testes and are commonly performed in surgical practice. These grafts create an aesthetically suitable neoscrotum by conforming to irregular defects and contracting on healing, resembling the rugae of a natural scrotum. They also enable drainage of exudate throughout the healing process and allow the graft to take nearly 100%.[28,53,54] Consideration should

be given to suturing the spermatic cord or testes together in midline before reconstruction in an effort to reduce surface area, facilitate wound healing, and prevent development of a bifid neoscrotum. Caution is warranted, however, when the wound bed does not demonstrate healthy, granulating tissue or if the tunica vaginalis is significantly affected. Other disadvantages of using STSG are the labor-intensive nature of postoperative wound care and the fact that these grafts are insensate.[55] Furthermore, grafts carry the risk of tissue adhesion to the testes, which can cause contractures that inhibit the cremasteric reflex and make the testes vulnerable to environmental conditions and trauma.[56] Local skin flaps are, thus, often used for scrotal and perineal reconstruction when the remnant scrotum is insufficient for primary closure (**Fig. 6**).

Multiple techniques have been developed to close perineal wounds with myocutaneous flap reconstruction. As mentioned previously, the goals of reconstruction must be kept in mind: durable testicular coverage, function of the graft and testes, and cosmetic outcome. Furthermore, planning for such a surgical venture must involve careful consideration of patients' current anatomy, their functional abilities, and the potential consequences of sacrificing various normal muscle bodies. Popular approaches to reconstruction include vertical rectus abdominis myocutaneous flaps,[28] medial circumflex femoral artery perforator flaps,[57] and anterolateral thigh (ALTP) flaps.[58] Yao and colleagues[58] describe the ALTP flap as a relatively simple single-stage procedure with minimal donor site morbidity. Use of a medial circumflex femoral artery perforator flap based on the musculocutaneous perforators of the gracilis muscle have been reported.[59] In addition, case series outlining the creation of a posteromedial thigh perforator propeller flap,[57] gracilis myocutaneous advancement flap,[60] and a groin fasciocutaneous island flap[61] can be found in the literature. Mopuri and colleagues[62] describe the modified pudendal thigh flap as a "robust, reliable, and resilient" reconstruction and should be considered when cosmesis and function are a priority. Perhaps as a consequence of the multitude of repair procedures, no single method of reconstruction has emerged as the premiere surgical option. Choosing to perform a flap versus a STSG remains at the discretion of the patients and surgeons.

PRIMARY URETHRAL CARCINOMA

Primary urethral carcinoma is a rare malignancy accounting for less than 1% of all malignancies.[63] Primary urethral carcinoma is diagnosed when the

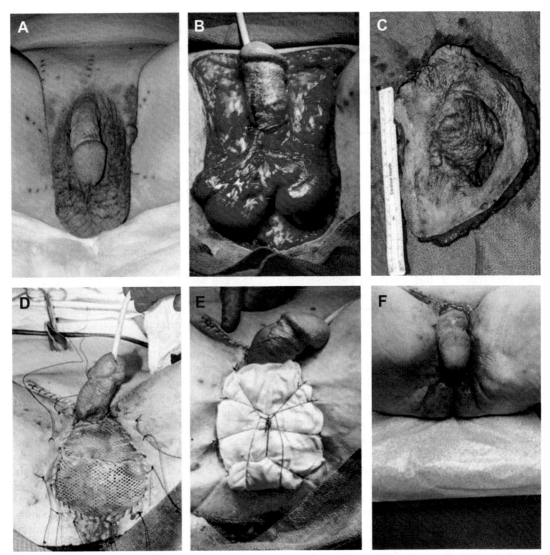

Fig. 6. (*A*) Preoperative appearance of a 79-year-old gentlemen undergoing wide-local excision of Paget disease affecting the scrotum, perineum, and pubic area. Scars from preoperative mapping biopsies can be appreciated radiating outward from the genitals. (*B*) Extensive local excision of all affected tissue created an approximately 15 × 18-cm defect. Note a ventral phalloplasty was performed and the penile skin was preserved. The testicles are seen in situ, sutured together at midline. (*C*) Surgical specimen includes the scrotum, perineal skin, and infrapubic area. (*D*) The defect was closed with fasciocutaneous flaps best seen in the patient's right inguinal area and a STSG of approximately 120 cm². The testicles were ultimately placed in medial thigh pouches before grafting. (*E*) The 0.18-in thick STSG was secured in place with a petroleum wound dressing bolster. (*F*) At 4 weeks postoperatively, the patient's wound was nearly completely closed. (*From* Beilan J, Baumgarten A, Mosiello G, et al. Mapping biopsies: a new tactic in the surgical management of extramammary Paget's disease. Video presentation: 111th Annual Meeting of the AUA, San Diego (CA), May 8, 2016; with permission.)

first carcinoma of the urinary tract is detected in the urethra, as opposed to secondary urethral carcinoma, which presents as carcinoma in the urethra after the prior diagnosis of carcinoma elsewhere in the urinary system.[64] For the purposes of this article, the authors address primary urethral carcinoma in male patients only. Various surgical treatment options for primary urethral carcinoma exist and include transurethral resection/fulguration, urethrectomy including distal urethrectomy only, and partial and total penectomy. Partial and total penectomy are discussed elsewhere in this article; therefore, the focus is on distal urethrectomy with reconstruction of the penis.

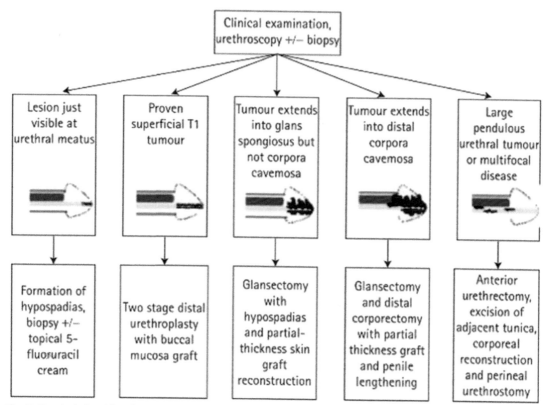

Fig. 7. Surgical algorithm for management of anterior urethral cancer. (*From* Smith Y, Hadway P, Ahmed S, et al. Penile-preserving surgery for male distal urethral carcinoma. BJU Int 2007;100(1):83; with permission.)

The goal in treating urethral carcinoma is to optimize functional outcomes and patient quality of life while maintaining oncologic outcomes. Surgical resection of urethral carcinoma should have a tumor clearance margin of 5 mm.[65]

Surgical resection of distal urethral cancer allows for reconstruction of the phallus, and Bird and Coburn[66] in 1997 were the first to report on phallus preservation for primary urethral carcinoma using a subcutaneous penectomy. This technique involves sparing the skin of the penis and the glans penis, mobilization and preservation of the neurovascular bundle, and excision of the corpora spongiosum and cavernosum of the involved segment of the urethra. Additional penile-preserving surgery for distal urethral tumors were highlighted by Smith and colleagues[67] and include hypospadias formation, buccal mucosa urethroplasty, glansectomy with corporectomy, anterior urethrectomy with excision of adjacent tunica, corporal reconstruction, and perineal urethrostomy. Smith and colleagues[67] subsequently developed a surgical algorithm to treat distal urethral cancers based on the tumor stage and grade, highlighting these techniques (**Fig. 7**).

The low prevalence of penile cancer, primary urethral cancer, and scrotal cancer in many ways presents a challenge for reconstructive urologists; therefore, many of the principles used in this domain are derived from techniques used in plastic surgery. In regard to penile malignancy, much is extrapolated from trauma patients and from sex reassignment surgeries. Urethral reconstruction is in itself its own subsect of urology, and many of the techniques used in penile and urethral reconstruction are used. Scrotal cancer reconstruction is derived from techniques learned in treating patients with Fournier disease as well as trauma and burn patients. The primary goal of any oncologic procedure remains oncologic control, but the goal in reconstruction in patients with cancer is restoration of form and function. This field is an ever-evolving field and continues to be a dynamic area of growth and potential for the urologic surgeon.

REFERENCES

1. Busby JE, Pettaway CA. What's new in the management of penile cancer? Curr Opin Urol 2005;15:350–7.

2. Backes DM, Kurman RJ, Pimenta JM, et al. Systematic review of human papillomavirus prevalence in invasive penile cancer. Cancer Causes Control 2009;20(4):449–57.

3. Hakenberg OW, Compérat EM, Minhas S. EAU guidelines on penile cancer: 2014 update. Eur Urol 2015;67:142–50.

4. Leijte JA, Kirrander P, Antonini N, et al. Recurrence patterns of squamous cell carcinoma of the penis: recommendations for follow-up based on a two center analysis of 700 patients. Eur Urol 2008;54(1):161–8.

5. Lont AP, Gallee MP, Meinhardt W, et al. Penis conserving treatments for T1 and T2 penile carcinoma: clinical implications of a local recurrence. J Urol 2006;176:575–80.

6. Windahl T, Andersson SO. Combined laser treatment for penile carcinoma: results after long-term follow-up. J Urol 2003;169:2118–21.

7. Shindel AW, Mann MW, Lev RY, et al. Mohs micrographic surgery for penile cancer: management and long-term follow-up. J Urol 2007;178:1980–5.

8. Brown CT, Minhas S, Ralph DJ. Conservative surgery for penile cancer: subtotal glans excision without grafting. BJU Int 2005;96:911–2.

9. Shabbir M, Muneer A, Kalsi J, et al. Glans resurfacing for the treatment of carcinoma in situ of the penis: surgical technique and outcomes. Eur Urol 2011;59(1):142–7.

10. Hadway P, Corbishley CM, Watkin NA. Total glans resurfacing for premalignant lesions of the penis: initial outcome data. BJU Int 2006;98(3):532–6.

11. Rohrich R, Coberly DM, Krueger JK, et al. Planning elective operations on patients who smoke: survey of North American plastic surgeons. Plast Reconstr Surg 2002;191(1):350–3.

12. Wells MJ, Taylor RS. Mohs micrographic surgery for penoscrotal malignancy. Urol Clin North Am 2010; 37(3):403–9.

13. Mohs FE, Snow SN, Larson PO. Mohs micrographic surgery for penile tumors. Urol Clin North Am 1992; 19:219–304.

14. Brown MD, Zachary CB, Grekin RC, et al. Penile tumors: their management by Mohs micrographic surgery. J Dermatol Surg Oncol 1987;13:1163–70.

15. Philippou P, Shabbir M, Malone P, et al. Conservative surgery for squamous cell carcinoma of the penis: resection margins and long term oncological control. J Urol 2012;188(3):803–8.

16. Ornellas AA, Kinchin EW, Nóbrega BL, et al. Surgical treatment of invasive squamous cell carcinoma of the penis: Brazilian National Cancer Institute long term experience. J Surg Oncol 2008;97(6): 487–95.

17. Yang J, Chen J, Wu XF, et al. Glans reconstruction with preputial flap is superior to primary closure for post surgical restoration of male sexual function in glans preserving surgery. Andrology 2014;2:729–33.

18. Palminteri E, Berdondini E, Lazzeri M, et al. Resurfacing and reconstruction of the glans penis. Eur Urol 2007;52:893–900.

19. Spiess P. New treatment guidelines for penile cancer. J Natl Compr Canc Netw 2013;11:659–62.

20. Belinky J, Cheliz GM, Graziano CA, et al. Glanuloplasty with urethral flap after partial penectomy. J Urol 2011;185:204–6.

21. Gulino G, Sasso F, Palermo G, et al. Sexual outcomes after organ potency sparing surgery and glans reconstruction in patients with penile carcinoma. Indian J Urol 2013;29(2):119–23.

22. Wallen J, Baumgarten AS, Kim T, et al. Optimizing penile length in patients undergoing partial penectomy for penile cancer: novel application of the ventral phalloplasty oncoplastic technique. Int Braz J Urol 2014;40(5):708–9.

23. Schultheiss D, Gabouev AI, Jonas U, et al. Bogoraz (1874-1952): pioneer of phalloplasty and penile implant surgery. J Sex Med 2005;2:139–46.

24. Garaffa G, Raheem AA, Christopher NA. Total phallic reconstruction after penile amputation for carcinoma. BJU Int 2009;104:852–6.

25. Garaffa G, Gentile V, Antonini G, et al. Penile reconstruction in the male. Arab J Urol 2013;11:267–71.

26. Hage JJ, De Graaf FH. Addressing the ideal requirements by free flap phalloplasty some reflections on refinements of technique. Microsurgery 1993;14(9): 592–8.

27. Monstrey S, Hoebeke P, Selvaggi G, et al. Penile reconstruction: is the radial forearm flap really the standard technique? Plast Reconstr Surg 2009; 124:510–8.

28. Salgado CJ, Monstrey S, Hoebeke P, et al. Reconstruction of the penis after surgery. Urol Clin North Am 2010;37:379–401.

29. Vriens J, Acosta R, Soutar DS. Recovery of sensation in the radial forearm free flap in oral reconstruction. Plast Reconstr Surg 1996;98:649–56.

30. Selvaggi G, Monstrey S, Hoebeke P, et al. Donor site morbidity of the radial forearm free flap after 125 phalloplasties in gender identity disorder. Plast Reconstr Surg 2007;118:1171–7.

31. Sengezer M, Oztürk S, Deveci M, et al. Long term follow up of total penile reconstruction with sensate osteocutaneous free fibula flap in 18 biological male patients. Plast Reconstr Surg 2004;114(2): 439–50.

32. Kim SK, Kim TH, Yang JI, et al. The etiology and treatment of the softened phallus after the radial forearm osteocutaneous free flap phalloplasty. Arch Plast Surg 2012;39(4):390–6.

33. Perovic SV, Djinovic R, Bumbasirevic M, et al. Total phalloplasty using a musculocutaneous latissimus dorsi flap. BJU Int 2007;100:899–905.

34. Djordjevic ML, Bumbasirevic MZ, Vukovic PM. Musculocutaneous latissimus dorsi free transfer flap for

total phalloplasty in children. J Pediatr Urol 2006;2: 333–9.

35. Selvaggi G, Monstrey S, Ceulemans P, et al. Genital sensitivity after sex reassignment surgery in transsexual patients. Ann Plast Surg 2007;58:427–33.

36. Zuckerman J, Smentkowski K, Gilbert D, et al. Penile prosthesis implantation in patients with a history of total phallic construction. J Sex Med 2015;12: 2485–91.

37. Hoebeke P, Decaestecker K, Beysens M, et al. Erectile implants in female to male transsexuals: our experience in 129 patients. Eur Urol 2010;57:334–41.

38. Mason C, Dunnill P. A brief definition of regenerative medicine. Regen Med 2008;3(1):1–5.

39. Zhang C, Murphy S, Atala A. Regenerative medicine in urology. Semin Pediatr Surg 2014;23:106–11.

40. Patel MN, Atala A. Tissue engineering of the penis. ScientificWorldJournal 2011;11:2567–78.

41. Kwon TG, Yoo JJ, Atala A. Autologous penile corpora cavernosa replacement using tissue engineering techniques. J Urol 2002;168:1754–8.

42. Chen KL, Eberli D, Yoo JJ, et al. Bioengineered corporal tissue for structural and functional restoration of the penis. Proc Natl Acad Sci U S A 2010; 107:3346–50.

43. Hu W, Lu J, Zhang L, et al. A preliminary report of penile transplantation. Eur Urol 2006;50:851–3.

44. Bateman C. World's first successful penis transplant at Tygerberg hospital. S Afr Med J 2015;105(4):251–2.

45. Tuffaha S, Sacks JM, Shores JT, et al. Using the dorsal, cavernosal, and external pudendal arteries for penile transplantation: technical considerations and perfusion territories. Plast Reconstr Surg 2014; 134(1):111–9.

46. Wright JL, Morgan TM, Lin DW. Primary scrotal cancer: disease characteristics and increasing incidence. Urology 2008;72(5):1139–43.

47. Morey AF, Rozanski TA. Genital and lower urinary tract trauma. In: Wein AR, Kavoussi LR, Novick AC, et al, editors. Campbell-Walsh Urology. 9th edition. Philadelphia: WB Saunders; 2007. p. 2649–62.

48. Por YC, Tan BK, Hong SW, et al. Use of the scrotal remnant as a tissue-expanding musculocutaneous flap for scrotal reconstruction in Paget's disease. Ann Plast Surg 2003;51(2):155–60.

49. Tiwari IN, Seth HP, Mehdiratta KS. Reconstruction of the scrotum by thigh flaps. Plast Reconstr Surg 1980;66(4):605–7.

50. Demir Y, Aktepe F, Kandal S, et al. The effect of scrotal reconstruction with skin flaps and skin grafts on testicular function. Ann Plast Surg 2012;68(3): 308–13.

51. Wang D, Zheng H, Deng F. Spermatogenesis after scrotal reconstruction. Br J Plast Surg 2003;56(5): 484–8.

52. Wang D, Wei Z, Sun G, et al. Thin-trimming of the scrotal reconstruction flap: long-term follow-up shows reversal of spermatogenesis arrest. J Plast Reconstr Aesthet Surg 2009;62(11):e455–6.

53. Mutaf M, Isik D, Bulut O, et al. A true one-stage non-microsurgical technique for total phallic reconstruction. Ann Plast Surg 2006;57(1):100–6.

54. Bryk DJ, Yamaguchi Y, Zhao LC. Tissue transfer techniques in reconstructive urology. Korean J Urol 2015;56(7):478–86.

55. Karacal N, Livaoglu M, Kutlu N, et al. Scrotum reconstruction with neurovascular pedicled pudendal thigh flaps. Urology 2007;70(1):170–2.

56. Atik B, Tan O, Ceylan K, et al. Reconstruction of wide scrotal defect using super thin groin flap. Urology 2006;68(2):419–22.

57. Scaglioni MF, Enrique Carrillo Jimenez L, Kuo YR, et al. Pedicled posteromedial thigh (PMT) flap: a new alternative for groin defect reconstruction. Microsurgery 2015. [Epub ahead of print].

58. Yao H, Zheng D, Wen J, et al. Reconstruction of major scrotal defects by anterolateral thigh flap. Cell Biochem Biophys 2014;70(2):1331–5.

59. Hallock GG. Scrotal reconstruction following Fournier gangrene using the medial circumflex femoral artery perforator flap. Ann Plast Surg 2006;57(3): 333–5.

60. Hsu H, Lin CM, Sun TB, et al. Unilateral gracilis myofasciocutaneous advancement flap for single stage reconstruction of scrotal and perineal defects. J Plast Reconstr Aesthet Surg 2007;60(9): 1055–9.

61. Aydin T, Feyzi K, Tayfun T, et al. Reconstruction of wide scrotal defect using groin fasciocutaneous island flap combined with a strip of deep fascia. J Plast Reconstr Aesthet Surg 2010;63(8):1394–5.

62. Mopuri N, O'Connor EF, Iwuagwu FC, et al. Scrotal reconstruction with modified pudendal thigh flaps. J Plast Reconstr Aesthet Surg 2016;69(2):278–83.

63. Gatta G, van der Zwan JM, Casali PG, et al, RARECARE working group. Rare cancers are not so rare: the rare cancer burden in Europe. Eur J Cancer 2011;47(17):2493–511.

64. Gakis G, Witjes JA, Compérat E, et al. EAU guidelines on primary urethral carcinoma. Eur Urol 2013; 64:823–30.

65. Minhas S, Kayes O, Hegarty P, et al. What surgical resection margins are required to achieve oncological control in men with primary penile cancer? BJU Int 2005;96:1040–3.

66. Bird E, Coburn M. Phallus preservation for urethral cancer: Subcutaneous penectomy. J Urol 1997; 158:2146–8.

67. Smith Y, Hadway P, Ahmed S, et al. Penile-preserving surgery for male distal urethral carcinoma. Br J Urol 2007;100:82–7.

Index

Note: Page numbers of article titles are in **boldface** type.

Urol Clin N Am 43 (2016) 561–566
http://dx.doi.org/10.1016/S0094-0143(16)30083-0
0094-0143/16/$ – see front matter

UNITED STATES POSTAL SERVICE®

Statement of Ownership, Management, and Circulation
(All Periodicals Publications Except Requester Publications)

1. Publication Title	2. Publication Number	3. Filing Date
UROLOGIC CLINICS OF NORTH AMERICA	000 – 711	9/18/2016

4. Issue Frequency	5. Number of Issues Published Annually	6. Annual Subscription Price
FEB, MAY, AUG, NOV	4	$355

7. Complete Mailing Address of Known Office of Publication (Not printer) (Street, city, county, state, and ZIP+4®)

ELSEVIER INC.
360 PARK AVENUE SOUTH
NEW YORK, NY 10010-1710

Contact Person
STEPHEN R. BUSHING

Telephone (Include area code)
215-239-3688

8. Complete Mailing Address of Headquarters or General Business Office of Publisher (Not printer)

ELSEVIER INC.
360 PARK AVENUE SOUTH
NEW YORK, NY 10010-1710

9. Full Names and Complete Mailing Addresses of Publisher, Editor, and Managing Editor (Do not leave blank)

Publisher (Name and complete mailing address)

ADRIANNE BRIGIDO, ELSEVIER INC.
1600 JOHN F KENNEDY BLVD. SUITE 1800
PHILADELPHIA, PA 19103-2899

Editor (Name and complete mailing address)

KERRY HOLLAND, ELSEVIER INC.
1600 JOHN F KENNEDY BLVD. SUITE 1800
PHILADELPHIA, PA 19103-2899

Managing Editor (Name and complete mailing address)

PATRICK MANLEY, ELSEVIER INC.
1600 JOHN F KENNEDY BLVD. SUITE 1800
PHILADELPHIA, PA 19103-2899

10. Owner (Do not leave blank. If the publication is owned by a corporation, give the name and address of the corporation immediately followed by the names and addresses of all stockholders owning or holding 1 percent or more of the total amount of stock. If not owned by a corporation, give the names and addresses of the individual owners. If owned by a partnership or other unincorporated firm, give its name and address as well as those of each individual owner. If the publication is published by a nonprofit organization, give its name and address.)

Full Name	Complete Mailing Address
WHOLLY OWNED SUBSIDIARY OF REED/ELSEVIER, US HOLDINGS	1600 JOHN F KENNEDY BLVD. SUITE 1800 PHILADELPHIA, PA 19103-2899

11. Known Bondholders, Mortgagees, and Other Security Holders Owning or Holding 1 Percent or More of Total Amount of Bonds, Mortgages, or Other Securities. If none, check box → ☐ None

Full Name	Complete Mailing Address
N/A	

12. Tax Status (For completion by nonprofit organizations authorized to mail at nonprofit rates) (Check one)
The purpose, function, and nonprofit status of this organization and the exempt status for federal income tax purposes:
☐ Has Not Changed During Preceding 12 Months
☐ Has Changed During Preceding 12 Months (Publisher must submit explanation of change with this statement)

13. Publication Title	14. Issue Date for Circulation Data Below
UROLOGIC CLINICS OF NORTH AMERICA	MAY 2016

15. Extent and Nature of Circulation			Average No. Copies Each Issue During Preceding 12 Months	No. Copies of Single Issue Published Nearest to Filing Date
a. Total Number of Copies (Net press run)			506	707
b. Paid Circulation (By Mail and Outside the Mail)	(1)	Mailed Outside-County Paid Subscriptions Stated on PS Form 3541 (Include paid distribution above nominal rate, advertiser's proof copies, and exchange copies)	200	278
	(2)	Mailed In-County Paid Subscriptions Stated on PS Form 3541 (Include paid distribution above nominal rate, advertiser's proof copies, and exchange copies)	0	0
	(3)	Paid Distribution Outside the Mails Including Sales Through Dealers and Carriers, Street Vendors, Counter Sales, and Other Paid Distribution Outside USPS®	154	198
	(4)	Paid Distribution by Other Classes of Mail Through the USPS (e.g. First-Class Mail®)	0	0
c. Total Paid Distribution (Sum of 15b (1), (2), (3), and (4))			354	476
d. Free or Nominal Rate Distribution (By Mail and Outside the Mail)	(1)	Free or Nominal Rate Outside-County Copies included on PS Form 3541	50	81
	(2)	Free or Nominal Rate In-County Copies Included on PS Form 3541	0	0
	(3)	Free or Nominal Rate Copies Mailed at Other Classes Through the USPS (e.g. First-Class Mail)	0	0
	(4)	Free or Nominal Rate Distribution Outside the Mail (Carriers or other means)	0	0
e. Total Free or Nominal Rate Distribution (Sum of 15d (1), (2), (3) and (4))			50	81
f. Total Distribution (Sum of 15c and 15e)			404	557
g. Copies not Distributed (See Instructions to Publishers #4 (page #3))			201	150
h. Total (Sum of 15f and g)			605	707
i. Percent Paid (15c divided by 15f times 100)			88%	85%

* If you are claiming electronic copies, go to line 16 on page 3. If you are not claiming electronic copies, skip to line 17 on page 3.

16. Electronic Copy Circulation	Average No. Copies Each Issue During Preceding 12 Months	No. Copies of Single Issue Published Nearest to Filing Date
a. Paid Electronic Copies →	0	0
b. Total Paid Print Copies (Line 15c) + Paid Electronic Copies (Line 16a) →	354	476
c. Total Print Distribution (Line 15f) + Paid Electronic Copies (Line 16a) →	404	557
d. Percent Paid (Both Print & Electronic Copies) (16b divided by 16c × 100) →	88%	85%

☒ I certify that 60% of all my distributed copies (electronic and print) are paid above a nominal price.

17. Publication of Statement of Ownership

☒ If the publication is a general publication, publication of this statement is required. Will be printed in the NOVEMBER 2016 issue of this publication. ☐ Publication not required.

18. Signature and Title of Editor, Publisher, Business Manager or Owner

STEPHEN R. BUSHING - INVENTORY DISTRIBUTION CONTROL MANAGER

Date 9/18/2016

I certify that all information furnished on this form is true and complete. I understand that anyone who furnishes false or misleading information on this form or who omits material or information requested on the form may be subject to criminal sanctions (including fines and imprisonment) and/or civil sanctions (including civil penalties).

PS Form **3526**, July 2014 (Page 3 of 4)

PRIVACY NOTICE: See our privacy policy on www.usps.com.

PS Form **3526**, July 2014 (Page 1 of 4 (see instructions page 4)) PSN: 7530-01-000-9931   PRIVACY NOTICE: See our privacy policy on www.usps.com

Printed and bound by CPI Group (UK) Ltd, Croydon, CR0 4YY

03/10/2024

01040304-0009